Best of Pflege

Mit „Best of Pflege" zeichnet Springer die besten Masterarbeiten und Dissertationen aus dem Bereich Pflege aus. Inhalte aus den etablierten Bereichen der Pflegewissenschaft, Pflegepädagogik, Pflegemanagement oder aus neuen Studienfeldern wie Health Care oder Ambient Assisted Living finden hier eine geeignete Plattform. Die mit Bestnote ausgezeichneten Arbeiten wurden durch Gutachter empfohlen und behandeln aktuelle Themen rund um den Bereich Pflege.

Die Reihe wendet sich an Praktiker und Wissenschaftler gleichermaßen und soll insbesondere auch Nachwuchswissenschaftlern Orientierung geben.

Nicole Adam

Pflegepersonen und demente Pflegeheimbewohner

Wissen, Einstellung und Pflegebereitschaft des Personals

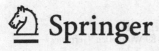

Springer

Nicole Adam
Graz, Österreich

Masterarbeit, Medizinische Universität Graz, 2015

Best of Pflege
ISBN 978-3-658-16335-8   ISBN 978-3-658-16336-5   (eBook)
DOI 10.1007/978-3-658-16336-5

Die Deutsche Nationalbibliothek verzeichnet diese Publikation in der Deutschen National-
bibliografie; detaillierte bibliografische Daten sind im Internet über http://dnb.d-nb.de abrufbar.

Gedruckt auf säurefreiem und chlorfrei gebleichtem Papier

Springer ist Teil von Springer Nature
Die eingetragene Gesellschaft ist Springer Fachmedien Wiesbaden GmbH
Die Anschrift der Gesellschaft ist: Abraham-Lincoln-Str. 46, 65189 Wiesbaden, Germany

Geleitwort

Die Pflege als eigenständige Profession und Wissenschaft leistet neben anderen Berufsgruppen im Gesundheitsbereich einen bedeutenden und unverzichtbaren Beitrag. Dazu bedarf es Pflegende mit umfassenden theoretischen und praktischen Grundwissen, so dass sie den derzeitigen und zukünftigen Herausforderungen im Gesundheitswesen angemessen gewachsen sind. Kennzeichen solch professioneller und qualitativ hochwertiger Pflege sind der Erwerb forschungsbasierten Wissens sowie dessen Implementierung und Anwendung in der Praxis.

Gerade in einer noch immer jungen Disziplin wie der Pflegewissenschaft ist es besonders notwendig, Forschungskenntnisse für die Praxis zusammenzufassen, wie beispielsweise durch die Ausarbeitung systematische Reviews. Dadurch kann der aktuelle Wissensstand zu einem Problem/Thema in übersichtlicher Form der Praxis zur Verfügung gestellt werden. Darüber hinaus ist es von großer Bedeutung, dass auch den gesellschaftlichen Entwicklungen und Bedürfnissen von PatientInnen Rechnung getragen wird und diese Aspekte frühzeitig in Aus-, Fort- und Weiterbildung berücksichtigt und entsprechende Inhalte adäquat konzipiert und vermittelt werden.

Eine entsprechende tertiäre Ausbildung und Qualifikation im Bachelor- und vor allem im Masterstudium der Pflegewissenschaft bietet hierfür die Grundlage.

Univ.-Prof. Dr. rer.cur. Christa Lohrmann
Medizinische Universität Graz / Österreich
Institut für Pflegewissenschaft

Institutsprofil

Das Institut für Pflegewissenschaft ist eines von 16 Instituten an der Medizinischen Universität Graz, Österreich und wurde 2006 gegründet. Angeboten werden entsprechend der Bologna Struktur Studiengänge für Pflegewissenschaft auf Bachelor-, Master- und Doktoratsebene:

Das Bachelorstudium Pflegewissenschaft in Kooperation mit dem Land Steiermark ist ein grundständiges, berufsqualifizierendes Vollzeitstudium (8 Semester) im Umfang von 140 ECTS mit dem Abschluss des Bachelor of Nursing Science.

Das modular strukturierte Masterstudium Pflegewissenschaft umfasst 120 ECTS und ermöglicht den Studierenden eine intensive Auseinandersetzung mit der (Pflege-)Wissenschaft. Es werden wissenschaftliche Kenntnisse und Methoden sowie die Möglichkeiten/Vorgehensweisen für die Umsetzung neuer wissenschaftlicher Erkenntnisse in die Praxis vermittelt. Daher liegen die Schwerpunkte über alle 4 Semester hinweg auf Forschungsmethoden/-techniken, Evidenz basierte Praxis sowie der Verbreitung und Umsetzung von Forschungsergebnissen. Das Studium führt zum Abschluss des Master of Nursing Science.

Das internationale Doktoratsprogramm „Nursing Science" wird gemeinsam mit der Universität Maastricht (NL) und in Kooperation mit der Berner Fachhochschule (CH) angeboten und dauert regulär 8 Semester. Die DoktorandInnen führen mehrere eigenständige Forschungsprojekte (i.d.R. klinische Pflegeforschung) durch. Die englischsprachige Dissertation muss 4 Artikel in internationalen peer reviewed Journalen mit dem/der Studierenden als ErstautorIn enthalten, in denen die Forschungsergebnisse veröffentlicht wurden. Die AbsolventInnen des Programms an der Medizinischen Universität Graz erhalten nach positiver Ablegung des Abschlussrigorosums den Titel Doktor/in der Pflegewissenschaft (Dr. rer. cur.) verliehen.

Das Forschungsprofil des Instituts für Pflegewissenschaft in Graz umfasst relevante Themen wie beispielsweise Pflegequalität, Mangelernährung, Inkontinenz, Umsetzung von Forschungsergebnissen, Pflegeabhängigkeit, Sturz, PatientInnenedukation uvm. Ergebnisse dazu werden umfangreich erfolgreich national und international publiziert und präsentiert.

Das Institut ist in Forschung und Lehre vielfältig national und international eng vernetzt. Es ist wissenschaftlicher Kooperationspartner für den gesamten Gesundheits- und Krankenpflege-Bereich in Österreich.

In allen Bereichen arbeitet das Institut nach dem Grundsatz:

„learning, teaching, research – joint effort for best care".

Medizinische Universität Graz / Österreich
Institut für Pflegewissenschaft
http://pflegewissenschaft.medunigraz.at

Inhaltsverzeichnis

Abbildungsverzeichnis

Tabellenverzeichnis

Abkürzungsverzeichnis

BIP	Bruttoinlandsprodukt
BPSD	Behavioral and psychological symptoms in dementia
CI	Konfidenzintervall
IG	Interventionsgruppe
KG	Kontrollgruppe
OECD	Organization for Economic Co-operation and Development
SD	Standardabweichung
WHO	World Health Organisation

Glossar

Agitation: ist das Zeigen von aggressivem Verhalten (Duden, 2013)

Apathie: Gleichgültigkeit gegenüber Anderen oder der Umwelt (Duden, 2013).

Bias: Ist die unbeabsichtigte Beeinflussung der Datenerhebung, der Datenauswertung oder der angewendeten Instrumente und kann zur falschen Interpretation der Ergebnisse führen (Bartholomeyczik, Linhart, Mayer & Mayer, 2008).

Inzidenz: Ist die Anzahl der Neuerkrankungen in einem bestimmten Zeitraum (Bartholomeyczik et al., 2008).

Median: Der Median liegt genau in der Mitte einer Datenerhebung. Dass bedeutet, dass 50 % der Werte größer und 50 % der Werte kleiner sind als der Median (Bartholomeyczik et al., 2008).

Mittelwert: Der Mittelwert gibt den statistischen Durchschnittswert bekannt. Er wird berechnet aus der „Summe der Messwerte, dividiert durch die Anzahl der Messwerte" (Bartholomeyczik et al., 2008).

Modus: Der Modus gibt an, welche Merkmale in einer Erhebung am häufigsten genannt werden (Eckstein, 2014).

Pflegeabhängigkeit: „Nursing care dependency is a process in which the professional offers support to a patient whose self-care abilities have decreased and whose care demands make him/her to a certain degree dependent, with the aim of restoring this patient's indpendence in performing self-care" (Dijkstra, Buist & Dassen 1998, p.146).

Prävalenz: Die Prävalenz gibt an, wie viele Personen zu einem bestimmten Zeitpunkt von einer Erkrankung betroffen sind (Bartholomeyczik et al., 2008).

p-Wert: Der p-Wert gibt die Wahrscheinlichkeit an, mit der die Nullhypothese abgelehnt oder ein Zusammenhang festgestellt, werden kann (Bartholomeyczik et al., 2008).

Rücklaufquote: ist die Anzahl der tatsächlich zurückgesendeten Fragebögen (Bartholomeyczik et al., 2008).

Standardabweichung: „ein Streuungsmaß für metrische Daten" (Bartholomeyczik et al., 2008).

Zusammenfassung

Hintergrund: Der demografische Wandel führt dazu, dass die Zahl der älteren Menschen ansteigt und dadurch auch die Demenz stetig zunimmt. Die Demenz kann zu Pflegeabhängigkeit führen, sodass professionelle Unterstützung benötigt wird. Pflegepersonen in Pflegeheimen sind mit BewohnerInnen mit Demenz oft überfordert, da ihnen demenzspezifisches Pflegewissen fehlt. Daraus resultieren zum Teil eine inadäquate Pflege sowie eine verminderte Pflegebereitschaft. Ausreichendes Wissen kann hingegen zu einer höheren Arbeitszufriedenheit und zu einer positiven Einstellung gegenüber BewohnerInnen mit Demenz führen.

Ziel: Das Ziel dieser Arbeit ist es, das Wissen über Demenz, die Einstellung und die Pflegebereitschaft von Pflegepersonen zu PflegeheimbewohnerInnen mit Demenz im Rahmen eines Literaturreviews zusammenzufassen.

Methode: Im Rahmen eines Literaturreviews wurde eine Recherche (Zeitraum: 2004-2014) in den Datenbanken PubMed, CINAHL, Embase via Ovid, Cochrane via Ovid, Gerolit und PsychInfo durchgeführt. Weiters wurde eine Internetrecherche in der Metasuchmaschine „Metacrawler" und „Google Scholar" sowie eine Handsuche in den Referenzlisten durchgeführt. Eine kritische Bewertung der Artikel wurde durchgeführt. Insgesamt wurden 16 Artikel inkludiert.

Ergebnisse: Pflegepersonen geben zum Teil an, dass ihnen Wissen über die Symptome der Demenz fehlt. Ihnen fällt es oft schwer den Schmerz richtig einzuschätzen und damit umzugehen. Durch Kommunikationsschwierigkeiten können Bedürfnisse oft nicht richtig wahrgeommen werden. Beim Erstellen eines Assessments fällt es Pflegepersonen schwer, Symptome richtig einzuschätzen. Die Einstellung der Pflegepersonen gegenüber Bewohnelnnen mit Demenz ist überwiegend positiv. Die Ausrpägung der Pflegebereitschaft ist nicht aussagekräftig.

Schlussfolgerung: Es sollten Schulungsprogramme angeboten werden um das Wissen zu vertiefen. Damit kann die Kommunikation zwischen BewohnerInnen und Pflegepersonen verbessert werden. Weiters sollten Pflegepersonen für Assessmentinstrumente besser geschult werden. Die Pflegebereitschaft von Pflegepersonen BewohnerInnen mit Demenz zu pflegen, sowie Zusammenhänge zwischen Einstellung und Wissen sollen erhoben werden.

Abstract

Background: The number of older people will rise because of the demographic change. Therefore the prevalence of dementia will increase. Dementia may lead to care dependency and professional nursing care is often needed. Care workers in nursing homes caring people with dementia are often unable to cope adequately, because of a lack in professional knowledge about dementia care. The result may be inadequate care and reduced nursing care preparedness. Knowledge about dementia care may lead to higher job satisfaction and to a positive attitude towards residents with dementia.

Aim: The aim of this literature review is to summarise the knowledge about dementia, the attitude and the nursing care preparedness of caregivers towards residents with dementia.

Method: A literature research in the databases PubMed, CINAHL, Embase via Ovid, Cochrane via Ovid, Gerolit und PsychInfo was made in the period of 2004 to 2014. An internet research in the meta search engines „Metacrawler" and „Google Scholar" together with a manual search in the reference lists succeeded. 16 studies were included and critically evaluated.

Results: In part care workers report a lack of knowledge about the symptoms of dementia. They have difficulties to assess and handle the pain of residents with dementia. Communication problems may lead to misperception of the resident's needs. In making an assessment care workers have difficulties to evaluate symptoms correctly. The attitude of caregivers towards residents with dementia is mainly positive. The intensity of nursing preparedness is not clear yet.

Conclusions: Caregivers should attend training programs about dementia care to deepen professionalknowledge. Thereby communication skills between care workers and residents could be improved. Nurses could be trained in using assessment instruments. In further research the care preparedness and the association between attitude and professional knowledge should be explored.

1. Einleitung

1.1. Demografische Entwicklung

Aufgrund der demografischen Entwicklung kommt es in den nächsten Jahren weltweit zu einer Zunahme der Bevölkerung. Die Weltbevölkerung im Jahr 2013 betrug 7,2 Milliarden Menschen und es ist zu erwarten, dass sie bis 2050 auf 9,6 Milliarden ansteigen wird. Dabei wird sich die Zahl der Menschen die 60 oder älter sind erhöhen. Es wird angenommen, dass es bis 2050 etwa zwei Milliarden und 2100 etwa drei Milliarden Menschen auf der Welt geben wird, die älter als 60 sind (United Nations, 2013).

Diese Entwicklung ist in Österreich ebenso zu beobachten. Laut Statistik Austria (2015) wird sich die Zahl der EinwohnerInnen in Österreich von derzeit 8,99 Millionen auf 9,37 Millionen bis zum Jahr 2060 erhöhen (Statistik Austria, 2015). Dabei wird die Zahl der älteren Menschen ansteigen. Derzeit sind 18 % der Gesamtbevölkerung in Österreich über 60 Jahre alt. Für das Jahr 2030 wird erwartet, dass 25 % der Gesamtbevölkerung die Altersgruppe der über 60-jährigen ausmachen wird (Statistik Austria, 2015).

Eine älter werdende Gesellschaft wird zukünftig eine große Herausforderung, sowohl für die Gesellschaft als auch für das Gesundheitssystem, werden (Eurostat, 2015). Gesundheitsprobleme nehmen mit dem Alter zu und die Häufigkeit und die Komplexität" der Erkrankungen sind bei älteren Menschen höher als bei jüngeren. (Robert-Koch-Institut, 2009).

Eine große Rolle im höheren Alter spielen psychische Erkrankungen, wie die Demenz (Robert-Koch-Institut, 2009). Kognitive Beeinträchtigung und Demenz sind weltweit die führenden chronischen Krankheiten, die zu einer Beeinträchtigung des täglichen Lebens (z.B. Kochen, Einkaufen, Waschen) und zur Pflegeabhängigkeit bei älteren Menschen führen können (ADI, 2013; Schüssler, Dassen & Lohrmann,

2015). Vor allem bei einer fortgeschrittenen Demenz ist der Grad der Pflegeabhängigkeit erhöht, sodass oft eine Aufnahme in ein Pflegeheim erforderlich wird (Marin, Leichsenring, Rodrigues & Huber, 2009; Schmidt et al., 2010). In Pflegeheimen können mehr als 50 % der BewohnerInnen von Demenz betroffen sein (Marin et al., 2009; Alzheimer's Association, 2014). In österreichischen Pflegeheimen weisen BewohnerInnen mit Demenz einen höheren Grad an Pflegeabhängigkeit auf als BewohnerInnen ohne Demenz. Sie benötigen Unterstützung in den Bereichen Hygiene, Kontinenz, An- und Auskleiden und Vermeiden von Gefahren (Schüssler, Dassen & Lohrmann, 2014).

Die Betreuung und Pflege von BewohnerInnen mit Demenz in Pflegeheimen ist eine große Herausforderung für Pflegepersonen. Häufige Verhaltensauffälligkeiten und psychologische Symptome der BewohnerInnen mit Demenz sind Depressionen, Angst, Agitation, Apathie und Aggression, die den Umgang erschweren und belasten (Bundesministerium für Gesundheit, 2006). Die Prävalenz von verhaltensbezogenen und psychologischen Symptomen (BPSD: Behavioral and psychological symptoms in dementia) liegt bei Menschen mit Demenz in der stationären Langzeitpflege bei 76 % (Ballard et al., 2001). Agitation, Depression und Aggression treten bei mehr als 50 % der BewohnerInnen mit Demenz auf (Ballard et al., 2001; Fauth & Gibbons, 2014), von Angst berichten 46,3 % der Betroffenen (Fauth & Gibbons, 2014). Diese herausfordernden Verhaltensweisen können bei Pflegepersonen zu emotionalem Stress führen, welcher Hilflosigkeit, Überforderung, Unzufriedenheit, Ärger und körperliche Bedrohung auslösen kann. Der emotionale Stress wird durch Faktoren wie Einstellung, Wissen, Erfahrung und Persönlichkeit positiv oder negativ beeinflusst (Höwler, 2008).

1.2. Wissen, Einstellung und Pflegebereitschaft

Pflegepersonen haben oft Schwierigkeiten mit dem Umgang von Personen mit Demenz, da häufig das Wissen über die demenzspezifische Pflege fehlt (ADI, 2013). Die Konsequenz kann sein, dass Personen mit Demenz eine inadäquate Betreuung oder Pflege erhalten. Darunter fallen z.B. das Ignorieren, Missachten, Nichtwahrnehmen der Bedürfnisse oder Vernachlässigen von vorhandenen Fähigkeiten. Pflegepersonen benötigen vertieftes Wissen über Demenz, um das Verhalten von BewohnerInnen mit Demenz zu verstehen und angemessen zu handeln (Sormunen, Topo, Eloniemi-Sulkava, Räikkönen & Sarvimäki, 2007). Wissensdefizite in diesem Bereich können zu Frustration, Stress und dem Gefühl der Unfähigkeit bei Pflegepersonen führen (Sormunen et al., 2007; Hsu, Moyle, Creedy & Venturato, 2005). Ungeschulte Pflegepersonen im Bereich der Pflege von kognitiv eingeschränkten Personen (z.B. Demenz) zeigen eine niedrigere Pflegebereitschaft als geschulte Pflegepersonen (Chang, Lin, Yeh, & Lin, 2010). Aufgrund von Wissensdefiziten werden vermehrt freiheitsbeschränkende Maßnahmen eingesetzt (Hsu et al., 2005).

Pflegepersonen mit ausreichendem Wissen über Demenz pflegen eher personenzentriert, berichten von höherer Arbeitszufriedenheit und einer positiveren Einstellung gegenüber PflegeheimbewohnerInnen mit Demenz (Zimmerman et al., 2005a; Travers, Beattie, Martin-Khan & Fielding, 2013). Eine negative Einstellung seitens der Pflegepersonen kann zu einer Verminderung von deren Arbeitszufriedenheit führen (Brodaty, Draper & Low, 2003). Aufseiten der BewohnerInnen mit Demenz ist eine positive Einstellung des Pflegepersonals verbunden mit einer erhöhten PatientInnenzufriedenheit, sozialem Wohlbefinden und einer Förderung der Gesundheit (Norbergh, Helin, Dahl, Hellzén & Asplun, 2006).

1.3. Demenz

1.3.1. Definition und Formen der Demenz

„Demenz (F00-F03) ist ein Syndrom als Folge einer meist chronischen oder fortschreitenden Krankheit des Gehirns mit Störung vieler höherer kortikaler Funktionen, einschließlich Gedächtnis, Denken, Orientierung, Auffassung, Rechnen, Lernfähigkeit, Sprache und Urteilsvermögen. Das Bewusstsein ist nicht getrübt. Die kognitiven Beeinträchtigungen werden gewöhnlich von Veränderungen der emotionalen Kontrolle, des Sozialverhaltens oder der Motivation begleitet, gelegentlich treten diese auch eher auf. Dieses Syndrom kommt bei Alzheimer-Krankheit, bei zerebrovaskulären Störungen und bei anderen Zustandsbildern vor, die primär oder sekundär das Gehirn betreffen" (Deutsches Institut für Medizinische Dokumentation und Information, 2014, p. 169).

Es gibt unterschiedliche Formen der Demenz. Die häufigste Form ist die Alzheimer-Demenz, sie beträgt weltweit 50-75 % (in Österreich: 60-80 %) danach folgt die vaskuläre Demenz mit 20-30 % (in Österreich: 10-25 %). Alle anderen Formen (z.B. Lewy-Körper-Demenz, Frontotemporale Demenz) sind seltener und machen höchstens 10 % aus. Auch Mischformen sind möglich (ADI, 2009; Schmidt et al., 2010). Folgend werden die zwei häufigsten Formen kurz dargestellt.

1.3.2. Alzheimer-Demenz

Krankheitsentstehung

Die Alzheimer-Demenz ist dadurch gekennzeichnet, dass im Verlauf der Erkrankung Nervenzellen in bestimmten Regionen des Gehirns absterben. Das Gehirn beginnt im Laufe der Erkrankung zu schrumpfen und es entstehen Lücken im Temporallappen und Hippocampus. Diese Gehirnareale sind für das Speichern und Abrufen von neuen Informationen verantwortlich (WHO, 2006; Grunst & Sure, 2010, S. 375ff; ADI, 2014).

Symptome

Die Alzheimer-Demenz mit ihren Symptomen können in drei Stadien eingeteilt werden. Das frühe Stadium wird oft übersehen. Verwandte und Freunde deuten auftretende Symptome oft als einen normalen Teil des natürlichen Alterungsprozesses. Die Betroffenen bekommen Sprach- und Gedächtnisprobleme (vor allem beim Kurzzeitgedächtnis), finden sich in der vertrauten Umgebung nicht mehr zurecht und haben Schwierigkeiten bei der Entscheidungsfindung. Sie können anspruchsvolle Alltagsaufgaben nicht mehr ausführen und das Interesse an Hobbys geht verloren. Es kann zu Depression, Antriebsmangel, Reizbarkeit und Stimmungsschwankungen kommen. Viele Betroffene sind in der Lage mit gewissen Einschränkungen den Alltag unabhängig zu bewältigen (WHO, 2006; Deutsche Gesellschaft für Allgemeinmedizin und Familienmedizin, 2008; ADI, 2009; Grunst & Sure, 2010).

Wenn die Krankheit fortschreitet, werden die Einschränkungen immer deutlicher (mittleres Stadium). Die Betroffenen haben Schwierigkeiten den Alltag zu bewältigen. Sie vergessen jüngste Ereignisse und auch Namen häufiger. Es wird bedeutsam schwieriger alleine zu leben. So sind viele Personen nicht mehr in der Lage für sich selbst zu kochen, die Körperpflege selbstständig durchzuführen oder einzukaufen. Die betroffenen Personen werden von Familienmitgliedern und/oder Pflegepersonen abhängig. Im weiteren Verlauf kommt es zu Schlaf- und Verhaltensproblemen (Umherwandern, Wiederholen von Fragen, rufen, klammern) und zu Halluzinationen (WHO, 2006; Deutsche Gesellschaft für Allgemeinmedizin und Familienmedizin, 2008; ADI, 2009; Grunst & Sure, 2010).

Das späte Stadium ist gekennzeichnet durch eine beinahe vollständig ausgeprägte Pflegeabhängigkeit und Inaktivität. Verwandte, Freunde und bekannte Objekte werden nicht mehr erkannt und der Weg zurück nach Hause wird nicht mehr gefunden. Es bestehen Schwierigkeiten in der räumlichen und zeitlichen Orientierung und der Kommunikationsfähigkeit. In der Öffentlichkeit können Personen mit Demenz ein

Verhalten zeigen, welches als unangemessen angesehen wird (z.B. sich Auskleiden). Sie benötigen Unterstützung in den Bereichen Körperpflege, Nahrungsauf-
nahme, Ausscheidung (Blasen- und Darminkontinenz), Mobilität (eingeschränkte
Gehfähigkeit) und An- und Auskleiden. Im Verlauf der Erkrankung werden sie vollständig pflegeabhängig (WHO, 2006; Deutsche Gesellschaft für Allgemeinmedizin
und Familienmedizin, 2008; ADI, 2009; Grunst & Sure, 2010; ADI, 2013).

1.3.3. Vaskuläre Demenz

Krankheitsentstehung

Aufgrund einer möglichen Herz-Kreislauferkrankung kann es zu einer Gefäßschä-
digung kommen, die wiederum zu einer Minderdurchblutung im Gehirn führt. Diese
verursacht einen Sauerstoffmangel und kleine Schlaganfälle können ausgelöst werden. Dabei sterben Gehirnzellen ab und dies kann zu Problemen mit dem Gedächtnis, Denken und der Merkfähigkeit führen (WHO, 2006; Grunst & Sure, 2010; ADI,
2014).

Symptome

Die Symptomatik und der Verlauf einer vaskulären Demenz sind bei jedem Betroffenen anders, da kleine Schlaganfälle unterschiedliche Bereiche des Gehirns und in
unterschiedlichem Ausmaß treffen können. Es kann zu Verminderung der Merkfähigkeit, Aufmerksamkeit und Konzentration kommen sowie zu Verlangsamung, Bla-
senstörung, plötzliche Verwirrtheit, Gang- und Sprachstörungen. Des Weiteren, vor
allem zu Beginn der Erkrankung, sind Depressionen, Stimmungsschwankungen
und Epilepsie möglich (Grunst & Sure, 2010; ADI, 2014; Bundesministerium für Gesundheit, 2014).

1.4. Inzidenz und Prävalenz von Demenz

Die Demenz ist eine der größten globalen Herausforderungen im Gesundheitswesen unserer Generation (ADI, 2013). Die Zahl der Menschen, die an Demenz erkranken, wird in Zukunft stark ansteigen. Im Jahr 2010 waren 35,6 Millionen Menschen weltweit von Demenz betroffen. Berechnungen zufolge wird sich diese Zahl alle zwanzig Jahre verdoppeln. Dies bedeutet, dass im Jahr 2030 etwa 65,7 Millionen und 2050 etwa 115,4 Millionen Menschen weltweit an Demenz erkrankt sein werden (ADI, 2014; Prince, Bryce, Albanese, Wimo, Ribeiro & Ferri, 2013; WHO, 2012).

Auch in Österreich steigt, aufgrund der älter werdenden Gesellschaft, die Zahl der Personen, die an Demenz leiden, stetig an. Im Jahr 2010 waren 90.500 Menschen von Demenz betroffen. Laut neuester Bevölkerungsprognose werden im Jahr 2050 in Österreich etwa 262.300 Menschen mit der Erkrankung Demenz leben (Schmidt et al., 2010).

1.5. Kosten

Demenz zählt zu den teuersten Krankheitsgruppen im Alter (Robert-Koch-Institut, 2009). Die internationale Alzheimervereinigung errechnete die jährlichen Kosten, die die Erkrankung Demenz verursacht, weltweit auf 606 Milliarden US-Dollar (Jahr 2010), die bis 2030 auf 1 117 Milliarden US-Dollar ansteigen werden. In Europa (2008) liegen die totalen Kosten für die Demenz geschätzt bei € 177 Milliarden. Von diesen Kosten sind € 96,6 Milliarden Kosten für die informelle Pflege und € 80,6 Milliarden sind direkte Kosten (Wimo et al., 2010).

Laut der Metaanalyse von Schmidt et al. (2010), werden die jährlichen Kosten für die Versorgung von Personen mit Demenz mit € 1,1 Milliarden berechnet. *„Etwa drei Viertel davon machen nicht-medizinische Kosten aus, während die medizinischen Kosten nur etwa ein Viertel betragen. Die Kosten, die durch die medikamentöse*

Behandlung entstehen, machen nur sechs Prozent der Gesamtkosten für die Versorgung Demenzkranker aus" (Schmidt et al. 2010, p. 71).

In Österreich werden, laut Berechnungen der Wiener Gebietskrankenkasse, die jährlichen Kosten für eine Person, die an Demenz erkrankt ist, in der häuslichen Pflege auf etwa € 12.000 und für die Betreuung in einem Pflegeheim auf etwa € 30.000 geschätzt (Grillenberger & Rossa, 2009). Für die Langzeitpflege in Österreich errechnete die OECD Ausgaben in Höhe von eins bis eineinhalb Prozent des BIP, das sind etwa € 3,1 Milliarden. Dabei ist zu erwarten, dass die Betreuung oder Pflege in einer Langzeitpflegeeinrichtung zunehmen wird und demzufolge muss auch mit einem Anstieg der Kosten für die Versorgung in einer Langzeitpflegeeinrichtung gerechnet werden. Die Ausgaben werden, laut Berechnungen, zwei bis drei Prozent des BIP bis 2050 ausmachen (Grillenberger & Rossa, 2009; Gesundheit Österreich GmbH, 2013).

Nachfolgend wird der theoretischen Bezugsrahmen der für diese Arbeit herangezogen wird, beschrieben.

1.6. Theoretischer Rahmen

Für diese Arbeit wird die Theorie „The theory of planned behavior" von Ajzen (1991) herangezogen. Diese Theorie versucht menschliches Verhalten in verschiedenen Kontexten vorherzusagen und zu erklären. Ein zentraler Faktor in dieser Theorie ist die individuelle Absicht (Intention) ein bestimmtes Verhalten auszuführen. Die Absicht hängt von drei Motivationsfaktoren ab, die einen indirekten Einfluss auf das Verhalten (behavior) nehmen. Diese Motivationsfaktoren zeigen die Bereitschaft ein Verhalten auszuführen an.

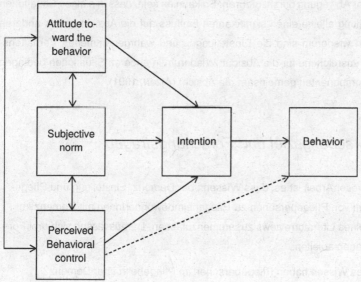

Abbildung 1: Theorie nach Ajcen (1991)

Der erste Faktor ist die „Einstellung zum Verhalten" (attitude toward behavior), der entweder positiv oder negativ sein kann. Der zweite Faktor ist die „subjektive Norm" (subjective norm) und ist ein sozialer Faktor. Er bezieht sich auf den wahrgenommenen sozialen Druck ein Verhalten auszuführen oder nicht auszuführen. Der dritte Faktor ist die „wahrgenommene Verhaltenskontrolle" (perceived behavioral control) und bezieht sich auf die wahrgenommene Leichtigkeit oder Schwierigkeit der Durchführung des Verhaltens und es wird angenommen, dass Erfahrungen aus der Vergangenheit sowie auch erwartete Hindernisse reflektiert werden.

Die Theorie besagt, dass je positiver die Einstellung und die subjektive Norm bezüglich eines Verhaltens und je größer die wahrgenommene Verhaltenskontrolle (perceived behavioral control) ist, desto stärker hat eine Person die Absicht ein Verhalten unter Abwägung durchzuführen. So kann es sein, dass in einigen Situationen die Einstellung alleine einen signifikanten Einfluss auf die Absicht hat. In anderen Situationen wiederum sind die Einstellungen und wahrgenommenen Verhaltenskontrollen ausreichend für die Absicht. Wiederum in anderen Situationen bedingen alle drei Komponenten gemeinsam die Absicht (Ajzen, 1991).

1.7. Forschungsziel und Forschungsfragen

Das Ziel dieser Arbeit ist es, dass Wissen über Demenz, Einstellung und Pflegebereitschaft von Pflegepersonen zu PflegeheimbewohnerInnen mit Demenz im Rahmen eines Literaturreviews zusammenzufassen. Daraus lassen sich drei Forschungsfragen ableiten:

1. Welches Wissen haben Pflegepersonen im Pflegeheim über Demenz?
2. Welche Einstellung haben Pflegepersonen im Pflegeheim über Demenz?
3. Welche Bereitschaft haben Pflegepersonen im Pflegeheim BewohnerInnen mit Demenz zu pflegen?

2. Methode

2.1. Design

Für die Beantwortung der Forschungsfragen wurde ein Literaturreview gewählt. Das Ziel eines Literaturreviews ist es, den aktuellen Wissensstand zu einem Thema zu erheben, dieses Wissen zusammenzufassen und zu evaluieren (Machi & McEvoy, 2012).

2.2. Ein- und Ausschlusskriterien

Einschlusskriterien waren, dass sich die Studien mit der Thematik Wissen und/oder Einstellung und/oder Pflegebereitschaft von Pflegepersonen zu Demenz auseinandersetzten. Als Setting wurden Pflegeheime als Einschlusskriterium gewählt. Auszubildende Pflegekräfte oder Studierende wurden ausgeschlossen. Limitationen bei der Literaturrecherche in den Datenbanken wurden in den Bereichen Sprache (englisch- und deutschsprachige Literatur), Zeitraum (2004 -2014), Suchfeld (Title/Abstract) und Auswahl von Forschungsartikeln gesetzt.

2.3. Suchstrategie

2.3.1. Datenbanken

Zu Beginn wurde eine Suche in der Datenbank PubMed durchgeführt, um wichtige Keywords zu identifizieren. Die Literaturrecherche fand in den Datenbanken PubMed, CINAHL, Embase via Ovid, Cochrane via Ovid, Gerolit und PsychInfo statt. Dabei wurden ausschließlich englische Keywords in Kombination mit MesH-Terms, Boolean'sche Operatoren und Trunkierungen verwendet. In der Datenbank Gerolit wurde mit englischen und deutschen Keywords nach relevanter Literatur gesucht. Die verwendeten Keywords sind in Tabelle 1 bis Tabelle 4 ersichtlich.

Tabelle 1: Keywords für Wissen

knowledge (Mesh) OR Professional Competence"[Mesh] OR know* OR competen* OR abilit* OR aware* OR expert* OR skill*

AND

Nurses (Mesh) OR Nursing Staff (MesH) Nurses' Aides (Mesh) OR nurs*

AND

Residential facilities (Mesh) OR "Long-Term Care"[Mesh] OR long-term care OR nursing home* OR residential

AND

Dementia (Mesh) OR dement* OR alzheimer* OR (cognitive* AND impair*)

Tabelle 2: Keywords für Einstellung

attitude (Mesh) OR attitude* OR belief* OR convic* OR opinion* OR perspective* OR position* OR view* OR think*

AND

Nurses (Mesh) OR Nursing Staff (MesH) Nurses' Aides (Mesh) OR nurs*

AND

Residential facilities (Mesh) OR "Long-Term Care"[Mesh] OR long-term care OR nursing home* OR residential

AND

Dementia (Mesh) OR dement* OR alzheimer* OR (cognitive* AND impair*)

Tabelle 3: Keywords für Pflegebereitschaft

"Motivation" [Mesh] OR „Job Satisfaction" [Mesh] OR motivat* OR will* OR read* OR engagement OR satisf*

AND

Nurses (Mesh) OR Nursing Staff (MesH) Nurses' Aides (Mesh) OR nurs*

AND

Residential facilities (Mesh) OR "Long-Term Care"[Mesh] OR long-term care OR nursing home* OR residential

AND

Dementia (Mesh) OR dement* OR alzheimer* OR (cognitive* AND impair*)

Tabelle 4: Deutsche Keywords

1.Forschungsfrage	2. Forschungsfrage	3.Forschungsfrage
Alzheimer ODER Demenz	Alzheimer ODER Demenz	Alzheimer ODER Demenz
UND	**UND**	**UND**
Langzeitpflege ODER Pflegeheim	Langzeitpflege ODER Pflegeheim	Langzeitpflege ODER Pflegeheim
UND	**UND**	**UND**
Pflege*	Pflege*	Pflege*
UND	**UND**	**UND**
Können ODER Fähigkeit ODER Wissen	Sichtweise ODER Einstellung	Bereitschaft ODER Motivation

2.3.2. Internetrecherche

Für die Suche im Internet wurden die Metasuchmaschine „Metacrawler" und „Google Scholar" herangezogen. Dabei wurde mit englischen und deutschen Keywords in den beiden Suchmaschinen nach relevanten Artikeln recherchiert. Es wurden jeweils die ersten fünf Seiten für die Suche herangezogen. Folgende Keywords wurden in unterschiedlicher Kombination verwendet:

Deutsche Keywords: Demenz, Wissen, Einstellung, Pflegebereitschaft,
                      Pflege, Pflegeheim

Englische Keywords: dementia, knowledge, attitude, preparedness to care,
                      nurse, residential, care home

2.3.3. Handsuche

Eine Handsuche fand in den Referenzlisten der bewerteten Artikel statt, um weitere relevante Artikel zu finden.

2.4. Auswahl der Artikel

Aus dem Titel musste hervorgehen, dass sich die Studien mit Wissen und/oder Einstellung und/oder Pflegebereitschaft von Pflegepersonen zu BewohnerInnen mit Demenz befassen. Anschließend wurde der Abstract nach den Kriterien von Polit & Beck (2012) beurteilt. Im Abstract mussten Hintergrund, Ziel, Methode, Ergebnisse und Diskussion ersichtlich sein. Die ausgewählten Volltexte wurden gelesen und überprüft, ob sie den oben genannten Ein- und Ausschlusskriterien entsprachen. Danach erfolgte die Bewertung der Artikel. Die Darstellung des Verlaufs ist in Abbildung 1 bis Abbildung 3 ersichtlich.

Metacrawler und Google Scholar

Zur Beantwortung der Forschungsfragen entsprachen 26 Titel den Einschlusskriterien, davon waren 20 Artikel Duplikate. Von den verbliebenen sechs entsprachen zwei den Kriterien und wurden zu den Volltexten hinzugefügt und bewertet.

Handsuche

Bei der Handsuche wurden bereits beim Titel die Duplikate aussortiert. Demnach wurden drei Artikel zur Bewertung des Abstracts herangezogen, davon entsprach ein Artikel den Einschlusskriterien, der Volltext wurde gelesen und bewertet.

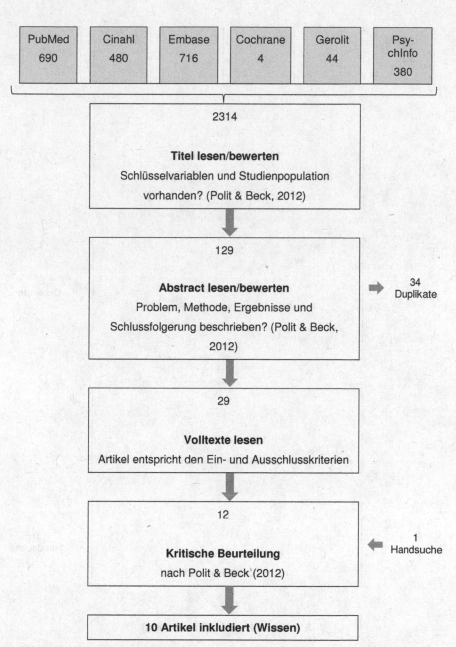

Abbildung 2: Flowchart zu Wissen

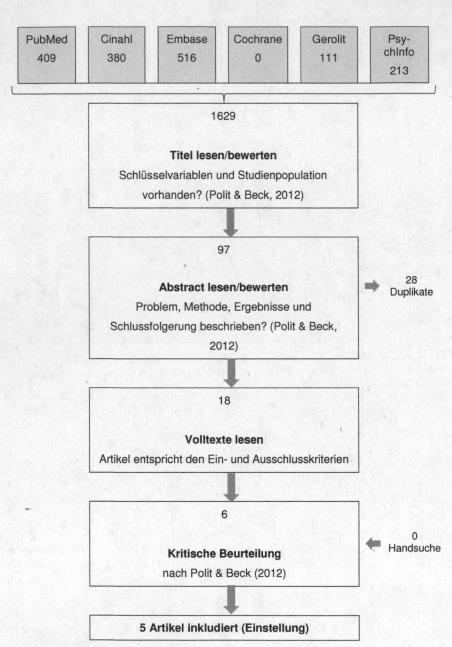

| PubMed 409 | Cinahl 380 | Embase 516 | Cochrane 0 | Gerolit 111 | Psy-chInfo 213 |

1629

Titel lesen/bewerten

Schlüsselvariablen und Studienpopulation
vorhanden? (Polit & Beck, 2012)

97

Abstract lesen/bewerten

Problem, Methode, Ergebnisse und
Schlussfolgerung beschrieben? (Polit & Beck,
2012)

28
Duplikate

18

Volltexte lesen

Artikel entspricht den Ein- und Ausschlusskriterien

6

Kritische Beurteilung

nach Polit & Beck (2012)

0
Handsuche

5 Artikel inkludiert (Einstellung)

Abbildung 3: Flowchart zu Einstellung

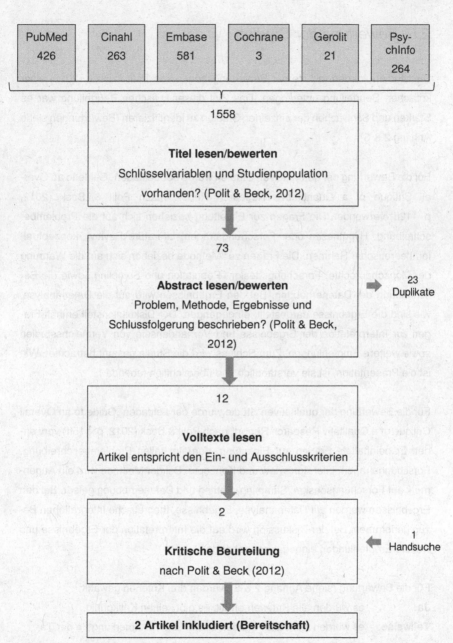

| PubMed 426 | Cinahl 263 | Embase 581 | Cochrane 3 | Gerolit 21 | Psy-chInfo 264 |

1558

Titel lesen/bewerten

Schlüsselvariablen und Studienpopulation

vorhanden? (Polit & Beck, 2012)

73

Abstract lesen/bewerten

Problem, Methode, Ergebnisse und

Schlussfolgerung beschrieben? (Polit & Beck, 2012)

➡ 23 Duplikate

12

Volltexte lesen

Artikel entspricht den Ein- und Ausschlusskriterien

2

Kritische Beurteilung

nach Polit & Beck (2012)

⬅ 1 Handsuche

2 Artikel inkludiert (Bereitschaft)

Abbildung 4: Flowchart zu Bereitschaft

2.5. Bewertung der Studien

Die Studien wurden mithilfe der Bewertungsbögen von Polit & Beck (2012) einer kritischen Beurteilung unterzogen. Das Ziel dieser kritischen Beurteilung war es Stärken und Schwächen der einzelnen Studien zu identifizieren (Bewertungen siehe Anhang 2 & 3).

Für die Bewertung der quantitativen Studien wurde der Leitfaden „Guide to an Overall Critique of a Quantitative Research Report" nach Polit & Beck (2012, p. 112ff) verwendet. Die Fragen zur Einleitung beziehen sich auf die Problembeschreibung, Hypothesen oder Forschungsfragen, Literature Review, konzeptueller/theoretischer Rahmen. Die Fragen zur Methode beziehen sich auf die Wahrung der Menschenrechte, Forschungsdesign, Population und Sampling sowie die Beschreibung der Datenerhebung. Bei den Ergebnissen wird auf die Datenanalyse, wie sind die Ergebnisse dargestellt, eingegangen. Der Diskussionsteil enthält Fragen zur Interpretation der Ergebnisse und Vorhandensein von Vergleichsstudien sowie weitere Empfehlungen. Zum Schluss wird die Studie gesamt betrachtet. Wie ist die Präsentation, ist sie verständlich und übersichtlich (ebenda.).

Für die Bewertung der qualitativen Studie wurde der Leitfaden „Guide to an Overall Critique of a Qualitativ Research Report" nach Polit & Beck (2012, p. 115ff) verwendet. Er beinhaltete Fragen zur Einleitung, darunter fallen Problembeschreibung, Forschungsfragen, Literaturreview und Konzepte. Bei der Methode wird ein Augenmerk auf Forschungsdesign, Sampling, Setting und Datenerhebung gelegt. Bei den Ergebnissen werden auf Datenanalyse, Ergebnisse, theoretische Integrationen Bezug genommen. Bei der Diskussion wird auf die Interpretation der Ergebnisse und weitere Empfehlungen eingegangen (ebenda.).

Für die Bewertung (siehe Anhang 2 & 3) wurden drei Kriterien gewählt:

Ja: es wurden alle Kriterien erfüllt, es gibt keinen Kritikpunkt.

Teilweise: es wurden nicht alle Kriterien erfüllt. Unter „Anmerkung" in der Tabelle ist eine Aufschlüsselung der Kritikpunkte ersichtlich.

Nein: Kriterien wurden nicht erfüllt / sind nicht vorhanden

3. Ergebnisse

Für die Beantwortung der Forschungsfragen wurden 16 Artikel herangezogen. Dabei befasste sich ein Artikel sowohl mit Wisssen als auch mit der Einstellung von Pflegepersonen zu PflegeheimbewohnerInnen mit Demenz.

3.1. Wissen

Es wurden sowohl Studien identifiziert die zeigen, dass Pflegepersonen Wissensdefizite zum Thema Demenz haben als auch Studien, aus den hervorgeht, dass Wissen vorhanden ist.

In der Studie von Hasson & Arnetz (2008) gab mehr als Hälfte (Einrichtung eins: 62 %; Einrichtung zwei: 54 %) der befragten Pflegepersonen (n=565) an, dass sie einen unzureichenden Wissensstand über Demenz haben (Hasson & Arnetz, 2008). In der Studie von Featherstone, James, Milne & Maddison (2004) konnten die Befragten (n=40) nur die Hälfte der 17 gestellten Fragen über Demenz richtig beantworten. Nach dem Schulungsprogramm konnten sie von den 17 Fragen 11,5 (Mittelwert) richtig beantworten. Aus der Fragebogenerhebung von Hsu et al. (2005) geht hervor, dass etwa ein Drittel der befragten Pflegepersonen (n=107) nicht wussten, dass Personen mit fortgeschrittener Demenz zu Aspiration und Erstickung neigen und sie gegen Abend hin verwirrter werden (ebenda.). Etwa die Hälfte (54 %) der Befragten (n=254) glaubte, dass Demenz ein normaler Part des Alterungsprozesses ist (Hughes, Bagley, Reilly, Burns & Challis, 2008). Weitere Studien fanden heraus, dass es Wissensdefizite über die Formen der Demenz und pharmakologische Behandlung, körperliche Symptome der Demenz und den Umgang mit demenzbezogenem Verhalten gibt (Chang et al., 2009; Furåker & Nilsson, 2009). Pflegepersonen (n=13) geben an, Schwierigkeiten mit demenzbezogenem Verhalten, wie Wandern, aufdringlichem Verhalten, körperlichen und verbalen Aggressionen zu haben (Chang et al., 2009). Ein gegenteiliges Ergebnis erbrachte die Studie von Robinson et al. (2014). Darin zeigten 85 % der befragten Pflegepersonen (n=174) vorhandenes Wissen über Pathophysiologie, Verhalten und psychologische Symptome von Demenz, allgemeine Entscheidungsfindung und demenzspezifischer

Pflege. Nach Hughes et al., 2008 erkennt die Mehrheit der Pflegepersonen (n= 254) die Symptome einer Demenz. Zugleich wussten 90 % der Befragten, dass Personen mit Demenz Familienmitglieder nicht mehr erkennen. 86 % der Pflegepersonen gaben richtig an, dass Vergessenheit ein Symptom der Demenz darstellt. Darüber hinaus wussten 82 % dass Personen mit Demenz nach Verwandten suchen, die bereits verstorben waren. Von räumlicher Orientierungslosigkeit der Betroffenen hatten 79 % des Pflegepersonals Kenntnis. 72 % der Pflegepersonen gaben richtig an, dass Agitiertheit ein Symptom für Demenz ist (ebenda.). Dennoch wussten 97,2 % der Befragten (n=107), dass das Kurzzeitgedächtnis verloren geht und das Langzeitgedächtnis bleibt. Weiters gaben alle (100 %) befragten Pflegepersonen richtig an, dass Demenz-Erkrankung in der Regel nicht plötzlich ausbricht (Hsu et al., 2005).

Im Bereich des Schmerzmanagements bei BewohnerInnen mit Demenz ist ein Wissensdefizit vorhanden. Schwierigkeiten bereitet dem Pflegepersonal (n_I=13, n_{III}=491; n_{III}=174) Schmerz von BewohnerInnen mit Demenz wahrzunehmen, zu bewerten und mit dem Schmerz umzugehen (Chang et al., 2009; Zimmerman et al., 2010; Robinson et al., 2014).

Ebenfalls Schwierigkeiten haben Pflegepersonen, wenn es um die Kommunikation mit den BewohnerInnen mit Demenz geht (Chang et al., 2009; Zimmerman et al., 2010). Pflegepersonen (n=22) geben fehlendes Wissen an, wenn es darum geht Signale von BewohnerInnen mit Demenz richtig zu interpretieren. Sie haben oft Schwierigkeiten zugrunde liegende Bedürfnisse von Personen mit Demenz zu identifizieren. Gründe liegen im fehlenden Wissen zu Hintergrundinformationen und in der Kommunikationsweise (Furåker & Nilsson, 2009). Das Pflegepersonal (n=22) hingegen stieß dann auf weniger Schwierigkeiten, wenn angemessenes Wissen verwendet wurde um verändertes Verhalten und die Körpersprache der BewohnerInnen zu identifizieren (Furåker & Nilsson, 2009). Die Mehrheit (83,2 %) des Pflegepersonals (n=107) wusste, dass das Diskutieren mit aufgebrachten Personen mit Demenz nicht hilfreich ist. Etwa Dreiviertel (74,8%) wussten, dass eine Person mit Demenz zwar sehen und hören kann, aber Schwierigkeiten im Verstehen und Begreifen hat (Hsu et al., 2005).

Ein weiteres Wissensdefizit besteht beim Erstellen eines Assessments (Chang et al., 2009; Furåker & Nilsson, 2009). Pflegepersonen (n=13) haben Schwierigkeiten Symptome richtig einzuschätzen. Dazu zählen Schmerz, Umgang mit Infektionen, Schluckstörungen und Verhaltensstörungen (Chang et al., 2009). Ebenfalls gibt es ein Wissensdefizit, wenn es darum geht, Zusammenhänge zu erkennen. Bei einer fortgeschrittenen Demenz fällt es Pflegepersonen (n= 174) schwer die Zusammenhänge von Delirium, Schluckstörung, Immobilität und Schmerz wahrzunehmen. Die reduzierte Mobilität wird fälschlicherweise nicht als Symptom einer Demenz erkannt. Dieser Identifizierungsfehler führt in weiterer Folge zu unangebrachten Interventionen und verschlechtertem Gesundheitszustand (Robinson et al., 2014).

3.2. Ergebnistabelle

Tabelle 5: Ergebnistabelle zu Wissen

Autor-/Jahr/ Land	Ziel	Population/Setting	Methode/Design	Ergebnis
Chang et al. (2009) Australien	Das Ziel war es, Herausforderungen zu identifizieren mit denen Pflegepersonen bei der Pflege von Menschen mit fortgeschrittener Demenz konfrontiert sind.	5 DGKS/P 4 PflegehelferInnen 2 TherapeutInnen 2 DirektorInnen oder StellvertreterInnen 10 Pflegeheime	Qualitativ: Action Research Daten wurden zuerst mit einem semistrukturierten Fragebogen und nachfolgend mit einem Interview gesammelt.	Herausforderungen: Umgang mit Symptomen und von demenzbezogenem Verhalten (Wandern, aufdringliches Verhalten, körperliche & verbale Aggressionen), Schmerzmanagement, Diagnose und pharmakologische Behandlung
Featherstone et al. (2004) England	Das Ziel dieser Studie war es, den Einfluss eines Trainingsprogramms auf Pflegepersonen zu evaluieren.	40 Pflegepersonen (20 Trainingsgruppe & 20 Kontrollgruppe) 2 Pflegeheime	Quantitativ: Pilotstudie Fragebogen: 17-Item Dementia Quiz um das Wissen über Demenz zu erheben.	In der Trainingsgruppe konnten Pflegepersonen im Durchschnitt 9,5 (Mittelwert) von 17 Fragen richtig beantworten und in der Kontrollgruppe 9,6 Fragen.

	Ziel	Stichprobe/Setting	Methode	Ergebnisse
Furåker et al. (2009) Schweden	Das Ziel dieser Studie war es, die Kompetenz von PflegehelferInnen, die BewohnerInnen mit Demenz pflegen, zu evaluieren.	22 PflegehelferInnen 4 Pflegeheime	Qualitativ 22 PflegehelferInnen schrieben Tagebücher und darauffolgend wurde mit 12 PflegehelferInnen ein semi-strukturiertes Interview geführt.	Defizite: Formen und Symptome von Demenz, Kommunikation mit BewohnerInnen mit Demenz und Erstellen eines Assessments. Kompetenz: Interpretation der Körpersprache.
Hasson & Arnetz (2008) Schweden	Ziel war es, die wahrgenommen Kompetenz, Arbeitsbelastung und Arbeitszufriedenheit von Pflegepersonen im Pflegeheim mit der Pflege zu Hause zu vergleichen.	565 Pflegepersonen: (24 DGKS/P mit Bachelor Abschluss, 354 DGKS/P & 187 PflegehelferInnen) zwei städtische Betreuungseinrichtungen für ältere Menschen	Querschnittstudie Einmalige Fragebogenerhebung zu vier Themengebieten: Kompetenz, emotionale und körperliche Belastung, Stress und Arbeitszufriedenheit. Antwortmöglichkeiten: „ausreichend", „unzureichend" oder „keine Ahnung".	In der Betreuungseinrichtung eins gaben 62% der Pflegepersonen an, unzureichendes Wissen über Demenz zu haben. In der Betreuungseinrichtung zwei 54% der Pflegepersonen.

Hobday et al. (2010) USA	Ziel war es, ein Schulungsprogramm für Pflegepersonen in Pflegeheimen zu implementieren und die Durchführbarkeit dieses Programmes zu überprüfen.	49 PflegehelferInnen 4 Pflegeheime 1 betreutes Wohnen	Quantitativ: Pilotstudie Fragebogen: "Dementia care knowledge" mit 15 Multiple-Choice Items.	Die PflegehelferInnen konnten vor dem Schulungsprogramm durchschnittlich 12,4 (SD=1,9) von 15 Fragen richtig beantworten.
Hsu et al. (2005) Australien	Ziel dieser Studie war es, das Wissen über mentale Gesundheit von DGKS/P (mit Bachelor Abschluss) zu identifizieren.	107 DGKS/P 70 Pflegeheime	Quantitativ Fragebogen: „Mary Starke Haper Ageing Knowledge Exam" besteht aus 25 Items zum Thema mentale Gesundheit; davon zehn Items über Demenz. Antwortmöglichkeit: „richtig" oder „falsch". Für jede richtige Antwort gab es einen Punkt und für jede falsche Antwort zwei Punkte. Score: 25 bis 50.	Fünf Fragen über Demenz wurden zu 80 % oder höher von den Befragten richtig beantwortet. Gesamter Fragebogen: Mittelwert: 38,36 Median 38 Modus 36

Hughes et al. (2008) England	254 Pflegepersonen 30 Pflegeheime	Quantitativ Fragebogen mit zwölf Items: Sieben Items befassten sich mit Symptomen von Demenz. Ein Item erhob die Sichtweise über Demenz und Altern. Vier Items bezogen sich auf Fallbeispiele. Für jede richtige Antwort gab es einen Punkt. Maximalscore: 12	<u>Kompetenzen</u>: erkennen von Symptomen (Vergesslichkeit, Agitiertheit, Wandern) <u>Defizite</u>: Etwa 50 % geben an, dass Demenz ein normaler Part des Alterungsprozesses ist und 10 % geben an, dass Kopf- und Gelenkschmerzen Symptome der Demenz sind.
Das Ziel war es, das Wissen und das Vertrauen von Pflegepersonen gegenüber PflegeheimbewohnerInnen mit Demenz, zu erheben.			
Pellfolk et al. (2010) Schweden	342 Pflegepersonen: (182 Interventionsgruppe & 160 Kontrollgruppe) 40 Pflegeheime (20 KG, 20 IG)	Cluster-randomisierte-Kontrollstudie Das subjektive Wissen wurde mit einer 100-mm-visuellen Analogskala gemessen. Score: 0 - 100 (wenig bis umfangreiches Wissen)	Die Interventionsgruppe erreichte einen Mittelwert von 70,6±18,1. Die Kontrollgruppe einen Mittelwert von 69,0±18,3.
Das Ziel war es, Wissen, Einstellung und den Einsatz von freiheitsbeschränkenden Maßnahmen vor und nach einem Schulungsprogram zu evaluieren.			

| Robinson et al. (2014) Australien | Ziel der Studie war es, das Wissen über Demenz von formalen Pflegepersonen und pflegenden Angehörigen zu erheben. | 174 Pflegepersonen: (35 DGKS/P mit Bachelor Abschluss, 36 DGKS/P & 161 PflegehelferInnen) Pflegeheime | Quantitativ Fragebogen: „Dementia Knowledge Assessment Tool version 2" um das Wissen über Demenz mit 21 Items zu erheben. Antwortmöglichkeiten: „zustimmen", „nicht zustimmen", „weiß ich nicht", „richtig" oder „falsch". Score: 0 – 21, je höher der Score desto größer ist das Wissen. | DGKS/P (Bachelor Abschluss): Mittelwert: 16,8 Median: 17 Range:11-21 DGKS/P Mittelwert: 16,3 Median: 16,5 Range: 11-21 PflegehelferInnen Mittelwert: 14,9 Median: 15 Range: 3-21 |

| Zimmerman et. al (2010) USA | Ziel war es, Wissen und Einstellung über Demenz und Verhalten von Pflegeperson gegenüber PflegeheimbewohnerInnen mit Demenz, vor und nach einem Trainingsprogramm, zu evaluieren. | 491 Pflegepersonen: (278 Interventionsgruppe & 213 Kontrollgruppe) 16 Pflegeheime | Randomisierten Kohortenstudie Erhebung von Pflegeleitbild, Kommunikation, Schmerzwahrnehmung und Umgang mit Schmerz. Für jedes Thema gab es einen Wissenstest mit jeweils fünf Fragen. Für jede richtige Antwort gab es einen Punkt (Score 0-5). | Mittelwerte für: Pflegeleitbild IG: 2,4 (SD 0,8) KG: 2,3 (SD 0,9) Kommunikation: IG: 3,2 (SD 1,0) KG: 3,1 (SD 1,0) Schmerzwahrnehmung: IG: 3,0 (SD 1,1) KG: 3,0 (SD 1,1) Umgang mit Schmerz IG: 3,5 (SD 1,1) KG: 3,6 (SD 1,1) |

3.3. Einstellung

Die Einstellung von Pflegepersonen zu PflegeheimbewohnerInnen mit Demenz ist durchwegs positiv (Kada, Nygaar, Mukesh & Geitung, 2009; Macdonald & Woods, 2005, Zimmerman et al., 2005a; Zimmerman et al., 2010; Gould & Reed, 2009).

Es wird dabei zwischen hoffnungsbasierter (hope attitude) und personenzentrierter Einstellung (person-centered attitude) unterschieden. Die hoffnungsbasierte Einstellung enthält Gedanken der Befragten über krankheitsbezogene Merkmale z.B. es gibt keine Hoffnung für Menschen mit Demenz. Hingegen beinhaltet die personenzentrierte Einstellung positiv gestellte Fragen z.B. Personen mit Demenz wollen respektiert werden, wie jeder andere auch (ebenda.).

Die Pflegepersonen (n=291) stimmten zu, dass es für Personen mit Demenz wichtig ist, dass sie das Gefühl haben respektiert zu werden, wie jeder andere auch (99,3 %). Zu einer guten Pflege zählt für 99,3 % des Pflegepersonals die Pflege von psychologischen wie auch von körperlichen Bedürfnissen. 97,3 % der Pflegepersonen finden es wichtig empathisch und verständlich zu antworten. Personen mit Demenz sind Menschen, die ein besonderes Verständnis brauchen um ihre Wünsche/Bedürfnisse zu erfüllen (95,2 % Zustimmung von Pflegepersonen). Sie stimmten auch zu, dass es viele Dinge gibt, die ein Mensch mit Demenz noch tun kann (94,2 %). Pflegepersonen finden, dass es wichtig ist, eine sehr strikte Routine zu haben, wenn man mit BewohnerInnen mit Demenz zusammenarbeitet (93,1 %). Weiters stimmten sie zu, dass Zeitverbringen mit BewohnerInnen mit Demenz sehr angenehm sein kann (92,8 %) und dass sie anregende und unterhaltsame Aktivitäten benötigen um die Zeit zu vertreiben (92,1 %). 81,1 % der Befragten stimmten zu, dass Menschen mit Demenz krank sind und betreut werden müssen. Mehr als die Hälfte der befragten Pflegepersonen gaben an, dass Personen mit Demenz eher zufrieden sind, wenn sie verständnisvoll und beruhigend behandelt werden (66,7%) und dass Menschen mit Demenz gute Gründe für ihr Verhalten haben (62,2 %). Etwa ein Drittel der Befragten ist der Ansicht, dass eine Person mit beginnender Demenz, eine unvermeidliche Verschlechterung erleben wird (31,3 %). Nach Ansicht von 21 % des Pflegepersonals seien Menschen mit Demenz unfähig Entscheidungen für sich zu treffen. 20,3 % sind der Meinung, dass es wichtig sei keine starke Beziehung mit

BewohnerInnen mit Demenz, aufzubauen. Für Menschen mit Demenz sei es wichtig, so viele Entscheidungsmöglichkeiten in ihrem täglichen Leben wie möglich zu haben (19,6 % Zustimmung). Etwa ein Zehntel der Befragten stimmten zu, dass Menschen mit Demenz Kindern ähnlich werden (13,1 %) und dass es keine Hoffnung für Menschen mit Demenz gibt (8,2 %). Ein geringer Teil stimmt zu, dass für Menschen mit Demenz nichts mehr getan werden kann außer die Grundbedürfnisse aufrecht zu erhalten (6,5 %). Kommunikation aufgrund der Vergesslichkeit der BewohnerInnen mit Demenz, spiele keine Rolle mehr (3,8 %; Kada et al. 2009).

In der Studie von Kada et al. (2009) kamen die AutorInnen zum Ergebnis, dass die Einstellung von der Ausbildung abhängen kann. Pflegepersonen mit geringer Ausbildungsdauer (z.B. PflegehelferIn) haben eine geringer hoffnungsbasierte und personenzentrierte Einstellung (p=0,02) als Pflegepersonen mit längerer Ausbildungsdauer (z.B. Diplomierte/r Gesundheits- und Krankenschwester/pfleger). Pflegepersonen mit zehn oder weniger Jahren an Berufserfahrung zeigen einen signifikant niedrigeren hoffnungsbasierten Einstellungswert als Pflegepersonen mit mehr als zehn Jahren Berufserfahrung (ebenda). Pflegepersonen (n=154), die zwischen ein und zwei Jahren Berufserfahrung aufweisen, berichten von mehr hoffnungsbasierter und personenzentrierter Einstellung als jene, die länger arbeiteten (Zimmerman et al., 2005a). Weiters zeigen Pflegepersonen, die zusätzlich eine Ausbildung in Bereichen wie Geriatrie, Psychiatrie, demenzspezifischer Pflege (Kada et al., 2009), Assessment oder Behandlung (Zimmerman et al., 2005a) hatten, eine höhere hoffnungsbasierte Einstellung als jene ohne Zusatzausbildung (Kada et al., 2009, Zimmerman et al., 2005a). Es konnte kein Zusammenhang zwischen personenzentrierter Einstellung und Zusatzausbildungen festgestellt werden (Kada et al., 2009).

Tabelle 6: Ergebnistabelle zu Einstellung

Autor/Jahr/ Land	Ziel	Population/Setting	Methode/Design	Ergebnis
Gould & Reed (2009) USA	Das Ziel dieser Studie war es ein Demenz-Trainingsprogramm in der der Langzeitpflege zu evaluieren.	71 Pflegepersonen 6 Pflegeheime	Quantitativ: Pilotstudie Fragebogen: Approach to Dementia Questionnaire (ADQ) zur Erhebung der Einstellung von Pflegepersonen über Demenz mit 19 Items. Score: 19-95. Ein hoher Wert bedeutet eine positive Einstellung.	Der Mittelwert liegt bei 77,8
Kada et al. (2009) Norwegen	Ziel der Studie war es, die Einstellung von Pflegepersonen zur Pflege von BewohnerInnen mit Demenz zu erheben.	291 Pflegepersonen: (75 DGKS/P mit (Bachelor Abschluss, 133 DGKS/P, 81 PflegehelferInnen & 2 k.A.) 14 Pflegeheime	Quantitativ Fragebogen: ADQ mit 19 Items (Score: 19-95) und beinhaltet zwei Domäne: • „Hope attitude". 8 Items (Score: 8-40) • „Person-centered attitude". 11 Items (Score: 11-55).	Gesamter Fragebogen Mittelwert: 70,3 „Hope attitude" - Domäne Mittelwert: 25,1 (SD 3,8) Range: 15-34) „Person-centered" - Domäne Mittelwert: 45,3 (SD 3,6) Range 34-53)

Macdonald & Woods (2005) England	158 Pflegepersonen Pflegeheime	Ziel war es, die Einstellung von Pflegepersonen gegenüber PflegeheimbewohnerInnen mit Demenz, zu erheben.	Quantitativ Fragebogen: ADQ mit 19 Items (Score: 19-95) und beinhaltet zwei Domäne: • „Hope attitude". 8 Items (Score: 8-40) • „Person-centered attitude". 11 Items (Score: 11-55). Je höher der Wert, desto positiver ist die Einstellung.	Gesamte Fragebogen Mittelwert: 75,86 (95% CI: 74,74 - 77,00) Median: 76 (Range: 49 - 90) „Hope attitude" Mittelwert: 28,53 (95% CI 27,92 - 29,16) Median: 29 (Range: 15 - 38) „Person-centered attitude" Mittelwert: 47,32 (95% CI 46,62 - 48,04) Median: 47,5 (Range: 34-55)

			Quantitativ	Gesamter Fragebogen
Zimmerman et al. (2005a) USA	Das Ziel der Studie war es, die Einstellung zu Demenz, Arbeitsstress und Zufriedenheit von Pflegepersonen zu erheben.	154 Pflegepersonen: (11 Administratoren, 1 DGKS/P mit Bachelor Abschluss, 1 DGKS, 136 PflegehelferInnen & 5 k.A.) 41 Pflegeheime	Fragebogen: ADQ mit 19 Items (Score: 19-95) und beinhaltet zwei Domänen: • „Hope attitude": 8 Items (Score: 8-40) • „Person-centered attitude": 11 Items (Score: 11-55). Je höher der Wert, desto positiver ist die Einstellung.	Mittelwert: 70,7 (SD 6,4) Range: 49 – 88 „Hope attitude" Mittelwert: 24,1 (SD 4,3) Range: 10 – 36 „Person-centered attitude" Mittelwert: 46,5 (SD 3,8) Range: 37-55
Zimmerman et al (2010) USA	Ziel war es, Wissen, Einstellung und Verhalten von Pflegepersonen über Demenz, vor und nach einem Trainingsprogramm zu evaluieren.	491 Pflegepersonen (278 Interventionsgruppe & 213 Kontrollgruppe) 16 Pflegeheime	Randomisierten Kohortenstudie Um die Einstellung von Pflegepersonen zu Demenz zu erheben wurde die Domäne „Person-centered-subscale" (11 Items, Score 11-55) des Fragebogen ADQ, verwendet.	„Person-centered attitude" Kontrollgruppe Mittelwert: 49,1 (SD 4,0) Interventionsgruppe Mittelwert: 49,0 (SD 3,8)

3.4. Pflegebereitschaft

In der Studie von Lee et al. (2013) gaben mehr als 90 % der Pflegepersonen (n=1047), die in einem Pflegeheim arbeiten an, dass sie bereit sind demenzspezifische Pflege durchzuführen. Es gibt eine Studie (Chang et al., 2010), die versucht die Pflegebereitschaft von Pflegepersonen (n=221) im Pflegeheim zu erfassen. Pflegepersonen mit drei Jahren Berufserfahrung weisen eine höhere Pflegebereitschaft als jene Pflegepersonen mit einem Jahr Erfahrung, auf. Pflegepersonen die noch nie Kurse zur Pflege von kognitiv eingeschränkten Personen besucht haben, zeigen eine geringere Pflegebereitschaft. Allerdings lässt der entwickelte Fragebogen keine Aussage über die Ausprägung der Pflegebereitschaft zu.

Tabelle 7: Ergebnistabelle zu Pflegebereitschaft

Autor/Jahr/Land	Ziel	Population/Setting	Methode/Design	Ergebnis
Chang et al. (2010)	Das Ziel der Studie war es, die Kompetenz und die Bereitschaft von Pflegepersonen über kognitiv eingeschränkte Personen zu erheben.	221 Pflegepersonen: (14 Pflege-Supervisor, 81 DGKS/P mit Bachelor Abschluss &126 PflegehelferInnen) Pflegeheime	Quantitativ Fragebogen „Preparedness of Caring for cognitively impaired elders scale". Besteht aus 10 Items mit einer 5-Punkt Likert-Skala. Score: 10-50. Je höher der Score, desto höher ist die wahrgenommene Bereitschaft.	Der höchste Mittelwert beträgt 3,22±1,07 (Item: Gestaltung der Umgebung) und der niedrigste Mittelwert 3,02±1,03 (Item: Ressourcen, Fähigkeiten).
Lee et al. (2013) China	Erhebung der Einstellung von Pflegepersonen gegenüber BewohnerInnen mit Demenz und ob vorhandene Programme die Einstellung beeinflussen können.	1047 Pflegepersonen Pflegeheime	Quantitativ Fragebogen besteht aus 4 Teilen: derzeitigm Stand (Prävalenz, Verfügbarkeit von Trainingsprogrammen), Meinung über demenzspezifische Pflege, Grad der Besorgnis von Demenzverhalten und demografischen Daten. Score: 0-5 (5 = sehr wichtig)	93,8 % und 90,4 % der Pflegepersonen sind bereit demenzspezifische Pflege durchzuführen.

4. Diskussion

4.1. Wissen

Das Ziel dieser Arbeit war es, ein Literaturreview zum Thema Wissen und Einstellungen von Pflegepersonen über Demenz sowie die Pflegebereitschaft von Pflegepersonen zu PflegeheimbewohnerInnen mit Demenz zusammenzufassen.

In drei Studien (Chang et al., 2009; Zimmerman et al., 2010; Robinson et al., 2014 wurde erhoben, dass es zum Thema Schmerz bei PflegeheimbewohnerInnen mit Demenz Wissensdefizite gibt. Pflegepersonen geben an, dass sie Probleme haben, den Schmerz von BewohnerInnen mit Demenz wahrzunehmen, zu bewerten und mit dem Schmerz umzugehen (ebenda.). Personen, die an Demenz erkrankt sind, sind oft nicht mehr in der Lage den Schmerz verbal zu äußern. Dadurch bleibt der Schmerz oft unbehandelt und die Lebensqualität der BewohnerInnen nimmt ab (Alzheimer's Australia, 2011; Corbett, Husebo, Achterberg, Aarsland, Erdal, & Flo, 2014). Der unbehandelte Schmerz führt zu Leid und Unbehagen und kann einen erheblichen Einfluss auf die Prognose und das Wohlbefinden jedes Einzelnen haben (Corbett et al., 2014). Das Review von Corbett et al. (2014) zeigt auf, dass Schmerz bei BewohnerInnen mit Demenz eine Verschlechterung der körperlichen und kognitiven Funktionen hervorruft, die Lebensqualität vermindert und die Lebenserwartung senkt. Weiters kann es zu einem erhöhten Sturzrisiko, Appetitlosigkeit und Schlafstörungen kommen. Die AutorInnen dieses Reviews merken an, dass Schmerz ein Faktor ist, der dazu beiträgt, dass einige Symptome der Demenz verschlechtert werden können (besonders Agitation und Aggressivität). So kann es sein, dass starke Schmerzen dazu führen, dass Personen mit Demenz weniger Herumwandern, jedoch das aggressive Verhalten gesteigert wird (ebenda.).

Eine verbesserte Schmerzbehandlung bei BewohnerInnen mit Demenz trägt dazu bei, dass die soziale Interaktion gesteigert wird, Verhaltensauffälligkeiten sowie kognitive und depressive Symptome hingegen vermindert werden (McAuliffe, Brown & Fetherstonhaugh, 2012).

Demnach wäre es von Bedeutung den Schmerz bei BewohnerInnen mit Demenz zu erfassen. Für die Schmerzerhebung können Assessmentinstrumente eingesetzt werden. Bei BewohnerInnnen mit Demenz, die sich im frühen Stadium befinden und sich verbal mitteilen können, ist eine Schmerzerhebung durch eine Schmerzbewertungsskala möglich (z.B. Visuelle Analogskala, Numerische Rating Skala, Gesichter-Schmerzskala; McAuliffe et al., 2012; Achterberg et al., 2013). Ist die Demenz fortgeschritten, sind Personen nicht mehr in der Lage den Schmerz zu äußern, die Lokalisation zu artikkulieren und verstehen die gestellten Fragen zum Schmerz nicht mehr (Achterberg et al., 2013). Anschließend sind Assessmentinstrumente zu wählen, die auf nonverbaler Ebene versuchen Schmerz aufgrund des PatientInnenverhaltens zu erheben (McAuliffe et al., 2012; Achterberg et al., 2013). Es wird von der US-amerikanischen geriatrischen Gesellschaft (AGS) empfohlen, dass Gesichtsausdruck, Verbalisierungen und Laute, Körperbewegungen, Veränderung der zwischenmenschlichen Interaktion, Veränderungen der Alltagsroutine, Veränderung des psychischen Zustandes bei der Erfassung von nonverbalem Schmerz herangezogen werden sollen (AGS, 2002). Es gibt unterschiedliche nonverbale Schmerzassessmentinstrumente. Sie unterscheiden sich hinsichtlich ihrer Reliabilität, Validität und ihres klinischen Nutzens (benutzerfreundlich, zeitlicher Aufwand, erforderliche Ausbildung; Herr, Coyne, McCaffery & Merkel, 2011).

Es gibt ein systematisches Review für Assessmentinstrumente zur nonverbalen Schmerzerfassung bei Personen mit Demenz. Dabei wurden sie hinsichtlich ihrer psychometrischen Eigenschaften und klinischer Verwendbarkeit überprüft (Lichtner, Dowding, Esterhuizen, Closs, Long, Corbett & Briggs, 2014). Es gibt zwar eine beträchtliche Anzahl von Assessmentinstrumenten, aber nur begrenzte Erkenntnisse über Reliabilität, Validität und klinische Verwendbarkeit. Für die nonverbale Erfassung des Schmerzes können Lichtner und KollegInnen (2014) keine Empfehlung für ein Assessmentinstrument im Pflegeheim abgeben. Dass solche Assessmentinstrumente noch weiter überarbeitet werden müssen und nicht für die Praxis geeignet sind, zeigten systematische Reviews von Zwakhalen, Hamer, Abu-Saad & Berger (2006), Herr, Bjoro & Decker (2006) und Herr et al. (2011).

Ein weiteres Ergebnis dieser Arbeit ist, dass Pflegepersonen Schwierigkeiten mit der Kommunikation mit PflegeheimbewohnerInnen mit Demenz haben (Chang et al., 2009; Zimmerman et al., 2010). Wissensdefizite werden seitens des Pflegepersonals geäußert, wenn es darum geht Signale und Bedürfnisse der BewohnerInnen richtig zu interpretieren. Pflegepersonen geben an, dass ihnen Informationen zur richtigen Kommunikation fehlen (Furåker & Nilsson, 2009). Durch den Verlauf der

Erkrankung wird es für Betroffene immer schwieriger sich verbal mitzuteilen und Probleme und Bedürfnisse nach außen hin zu zeigen (Bundesministerium für Gesundheit, 2006; ADI, 2013). Der Verlust der Kommunikation kann sowohl bei den Betroffenen als auch bei Pflegenden zu Frustration führen (Alzheimer's Australia, 2015). Die Kommunikationsfähigkeiten von Pflegepersonen zu BewohnerInnen mit Demenz können einen Einfluss auf die Lebensqualität haben (Zimmermann et al., 2005b; Vasse, Vernooij-Dassen, Spijker, Rikkert & Raymond, 2010).

In der Literatur findet man unterschiedliche Schulungsprogramme zur Verbesserung der Kommunikation. Das systematische Review von Vasse et al. (2010) nennt zwei Formen der Schulungsprogramme. Bei der ersten Form handelt es sich um strukturierte und kommunikative Einheiten, die zu festgelegten Zeiten stattfinden. In diesen Einheiten haben Pflegepersonen die Möglichkeit durch Einzelaufgaben (z.B. Lebensrückblick, Perspektivenübernahme durch Rollenspiel) ihre Kommunikation zu verbessern. Die zweite Form versucht Kommunikationstechniken bei der täglichen Pflege zu verbessern. Die nonverbale Kommunikation wird hierbei in der Praxis eingeübt.

Eine positive Wirkung für beide Schulungsprogramme wird in Einzelstudien nahegelegt. Sie verbessern die verbale und nonverbale Kommunikation bei Pflegepersonen als auch bei BewohnerInnen mit Demenz. Es wird sowohl die Zusammenarbeit zwischen BewohnerIn und Pflegeperson gestärkt als auch die Kommunikationsfähigkeit aufrechterhalten (Sprangers, Dijkstra & Romijn-Luijten, 2015; Vasse et al., 2010). Durch die Schulungsprogramme verwenden Pflegepersonen kurze Anleitungen und drücken sich positiv aus (Sprangers, Dijkstra & Romijn-Luijten, 2015). Nach Vasse et al. (2010) sollten Schulungsprogramme Zeit für persönliches Feedback und interaktive Lernformen beinhalten. Weiters sollten regelmäßige Auffrischungskurse angeboten werden.

Pflegepersonen in Pflegeheimen weisen einen unterschiedlichen Wissensstand über Demenz auf. Es werden Wissensdefizite über die Demenzformen (Furåker & Nilsson, 2009), Symptome der Demenz und den Umgang mit demenzbezogenem Verhalten angegeben (Chang et al., 2009; Furåker & Nilsson, 2009). Anderen Studien zufolge haben Pflegepersonen ausreichendes Wissen über Symptome der Demenz (Robinson et al., 2014; Hughes et al., 2008; Hsu et al., 2005). Dieses unterschiedliche Ergebnis kann möglicherweise durch das Studiendesign und den Grad der Ausbildung erklärt werden. Bei den beiden Studien (Chang et al., 2009; Furåker & Nilsson, 2009) handelt es sich um qualitative Studien mit kleiner Stichprobe, die überwiegend PflegehelferInnen befragten. Hingegen weisen die anderen drei Studien (Robinson et al., 2014; Hughes et al., 2008; Hsu et al., 2005) eine größere Studienpopulation auf und der Grad der Ausbildung ist höher. Pflegepersonen haben weniger Schwierigkeiten Verhaltensprobleme von Personen mit Demenz zu beschreiben (Robinson et al., 2014; Hughes et al., 2008).

Unzureichendes Wissen über Demenz kann dazu beitragen, dass häufiger freiheitsbeschränkende Maßnahmen eingesetzt werden und Medikamente für die Sedierung missbraucht werden (Hsu et al., 2005). Aufgrund der Wissensdefizite erhöht sich der Stress bei Pflegepersonen (Chang et al., 2010; Hsu et al., 2005; Edvardsson, Sandman, Nay & Karlsson, 2009) und beeinflusst die Arbeitszufriedenheit (Chang et al., 2010; Zimmerman et al., 2005a). Die Studie von Zimmerman et al. (2005a) fand heraus, dass besser geschulte Pflegepersonen von einer höheren Arbeitszufriedenheit berichten. Ebenso hat die Ausbildung der Pflegepersonen einen Einfluss auf die Arbeitsbelastung. Eine geringe Ausbildung kann ein Prädiktor für eine erhöhte Arbeitsbelastung sein (Edvardsson et al., 2009). In Pflegeheimen mit Demenz geht ein geringeres Ausmaß von verbalen Verhaltensauffälligkeiten mit einer niedrigeren Arbeitsbelastung des Pflegepersonals einher (Edvardsson, Sandman, Nay & Karlsson, 2008).

Des Weiteren kann unzureichendes Wissen zu einer inadäquaten Betreuung oder Pflege führen. Personen mit höherem Grad an Pflegeabhängigkeit erleben eher eine inadäquate Betreuung oder Pflege. Inadäquate Betreuung erfahren vor allem BewohnerInnen, die körperlich und kognitiv stark eingeschränkt sind (Sormunen et al., 2007). Dabei handelt es sich um Vorenthaltung pflegerischer Maßnahmen, Objektivierung (Behandeln der BewohnerInnen als Objekte), Ignorieren, Missachtung der vorhandenen Fähigkeiten und Infantilismus (BewohnerInnen werden nicht wie erwachsene Personen behandelt; Sormunen et al., 2007).
Wissensdefizite gibt es im Bereich des Erstellens eines Assessments (Chang et al., 2009; Furåker & Nilsson, 2009). Pflegepersonen fällt es schwer Schmerz, Infektionen, Schluck- und Verhaltensstörungen richtig einzuschätzen (Chang et al., 2009). Diese genannten Symptome betreffen vor allem BewohnerInnen mit einer fortgeschrittenen Demenz und werden oft nicht erkannt. Der Grund liegt auf der einen

Seite darin, dass sich die BewohnerInnen nicht mehr verbal mitteilen können und auf der anderen Seite, dass Pflegepersonen Schwierigkeiten haben ein Assessment zu erstellen (ADI, 2013). Das Pflegeassessment ist jedoch ein wichtiger Schritt im Pflegeprozess. Hierbei werden pflegerische Informationen gesammelt, die für die weitere Pflegeplanung relevant sind. Es werden die Pflegebedürfnisse als auch der Grad der Pflegeabhängigkeit erhoben (Alzheimer's Association, 2009; Bundesministerium für Gesundheit, 2010). Ein ganzheitliches Assessment von den Fähigkeiten und Hintergrundinformationen der BewohnerInnen ist notwendig um den BewohnerInnen eine individuelle und adäquate Pflege zukommen zu lassen. Ein umfangreiches Assessment beinhaltet die kognitive und körperliche Gesundheit, körperliche, sensorische und Entscheidungsfähigkeit, persönlicher und kultureller Hintergrund, spirituelle Bedürfnisse und Kommunikationsfähigkeiten sowie das momentane Verhalten (Alzheimer's Association, 2009).

Dabei sollte das Assessment Informationen enthalten, die von BewohnerInnen und Familienangehörigen selbst stammen. Ist dies nicht möglich können durch Durchsicht der Patientenakten und Beobachtung der BewohnerInnen Informationen gesammelt werden. Das gezeigte Verhalten der BewohnerInnen kann als Kommunikation verstanden werden. Vorlieben und Abneigungen können dadurch identifiziert werden (Alzheimer's Association, 2009).

Für eine weitere Informationssammlung können Assessmentinstrumente herangezogen werden. Das Ziel von Assessmentinstrumenten ist es, die Objektivität zu erhöhen und die Subjektivität zu verringern. Sie können als Grundlage für eine Entscheidungsfindung herangezogen werden. Ein Assessmentinstrument sollte valide und reliabel sein. Für die Validität wichtig sind hierbei die Augenschein-, Konstrukt- und die Übereinstimmungsvalidität. Die Reliabilität umfasst die Interrater- und die Test-Retest Reliabilität. Weiters ist es wichtig, dass das Instrument in der Praxis anwendbar ist (Bartholomeyczik et al., 2008; Sheehan, 2012).

4.2. Einstellung

Die Einstellung von Pflegepersonen zu PflegeheimbewohnerInnen mit Demenz ist in fünf Studien positiv (Kada et al., 2009; Macdonald & Woods, 2005; Zimmerman et al., 2005a; Zimmerman et al., 2010; Gould & Reed, 2009). Pflegepersonen fokussieren sich mehr auf personenzentrierte-Einstellungen (positive Merkmale z.B. Personen mit Demenz wollen respektiert werden, wie jeder andere auch) als auf hoffnungsbasierte (krankheitsbezogene Merkmale z.B. es gibt keine Hoffnung für Menschen mit Demenz; Kada et al., 2009; Macdonald & Woods, 2005; Zimmerman et al., 2005a). Die Einstellung von Pflegepersonen zu PflegeheimbewohnerInnen mit Demenz, kann mit der Ausbildung und dem Wissensstand zusammenhängen. Pflegepersonen, die Wissen über Demenz verfügen, haben eher eine positive Einstellung gegenüber BewohnerInnen mit Demenz (Travers et al., 2013, Kada et al., 2009; Hsu et al., 2004; Richardson, Kitchen & Livingston, 2002). Pflegepersonen mit einer Fachausbildung zum Thema Demenz zeigen eine bedeutsam höhere hoffnungsbasierte Einstellung (Kada et al., 2009).

Pflegepersonen, die PatientInnen als wertlos betrachten, sehen die Fürsorge für die PatientInnen eher als wertlos und ihre pflegerische Tätigkeiten eher als bedeutungslos an (Norbergh et al., 2006). Die Einstellung von Pflegepersonen ist für die Qualität der Betreuung und Pflege bedeutsam. Eine positive Einstellung führt zu einem Verhalten, welches die Patientenzufriedenheit erhöht und die Gesundheit fördert (ebenda). Es gibt Studien die nahelegen, dass eine positive Einstellung gegenüber PflegeheimbewohnerInnen mit Demenz, positive Auswirkungen sowohl auf Pflegepersonen als auch auf BewohnerInnen haben (Travers et al., 2013; Edvardsson et al., 2008). In der Studie von Travers et al. (2013) kamen die AutorInnen zum Ergebnis, dass eine positive Einstellung von Pflegepersonen gegenüber BewohnerInnen mit Demenz dazu führt, dass das Verhalten seitens der Pflegepersonen positiv ist. Außerdem kann eine positive Einstellung zu einer verbesserten Lebensqualität beitragen und bei Pflegepersonen zu mehr Engagement führen. Des Weiteren kann ein positives Pflegeklima die Prävalenz von Weglauftendenzen, Wandern und aggressiven Verhaltensweisen signifikant reduzieren (Edwardsson et al., 2008). Hingegen ist eine negative Einstellung gegenüber BewohnerInnen assoziiert mit weniger Arbeitszufriedenheit (Brodaty et al., 2003).

4.3. Pflegebereitschaft

Die Pflegebereitschaft von Pflegepersonen zu BewohnerInnen mit Demenz wird nur in zwei Studien erhoben. In der Studie von Lee et al. (2013) waren Pflegepersonen, die in einem Pflegeheim arbeiteten, bereit BewohnerInnen mit Demenz zu pflegen. Die Bereitschaft kann von der Berufserfahrung abhängig sein. Pflegepersonen mit drei Jahren Berufserfahrung haben eine höhere Bereitschaft als jene mit einem Jahr Erfahrung. Pflegepersonen, die noch nie Kurse besucht hatten, in denen es um die Pflege von kognitiv eingeschränkten Personen geht, zeigten eine geringere Pflegebereitschaft (Chang et al., 2010).

Die höhere Pflegebereitschaft bei Pflegepersonen mit längerer Berufserfahrung könnte zum Teil auf erhöhtes Wissen zurückzuführen sein. Dabei kann das Wissen einerseits durch Fortbildungen erworben worden sein andererseits durch Erfahrung (Erfahrungswissen). Pflegepersonen mit mehr als drei Jahren Berufserfahrung können mit Situationen anders umgehen als Pflegepersonen mit weniger Berufserfahrung. Erfahrene Pflegende können die gesamte Situation schnell und genauer erfassen. Sie können auf Erfahrungen früherer Pflegesituationen zurückgreifen und spontan reagieren. Sie sind in der Lage aus einer Pflegesituation die wichtigsten Aspekte zu erfassen und damit können sie das eigentliche Problem schneller erkennen. Durch die längere Berufserfahrung arbeiten Pflegende organisierter und effizienter. Des Weiteren entwickelt sich ein Gefühl der Kompetenz (Brenner, 1994). Durch die entwickelte Fachkompetenz sind Pflegepersonen in der Lage *"Aufgaben und Probleme zielorientiert, sachgerecht, methodengeleitet und selbstständig zu lösen und das Ergebnis zu beurteilen"* (KMK, 2011, p. 15). Womöglich spielt diese Fachkompetenz mitunter eine Rolle für die Pflegebereitschaft. Durch die längere Berufserfahrung wäre es denkbar, dass sich in dieser Zeit die Einstellung der Pflegepersonen gegenüber BewohnerInnen mit Demenz verändert und die Pflegebereitschaft positiv beeinflusst hat. Die Einstellung könnte wiederum mit dem Fachwissen zusammenhängen. Wie aus den Studie Zimmerman et al. (2005a) und Travers et al. (2013) ersichtlich, kann ausreichendes Wissen einen positiven Einfluss auf die Einstellung haben. Ebenso wäre es möglich, dass durch Erfahrungen die Einstellung verändert werden kann (Mamerow, 2006; Martens, 2009).

4.4. Theoretischer Bezugsrahmen

Die Theorie nach Ajzen (1999), die versucht menschliches Verhalten vorherzusagen, kann für die Beantwortung der Forschungsfragen herangezogen werden.

Die Theorie geht davon aus, dass die „Einstellung gegenüber einem Verhalten" (positiv oder negativ), die „subjektive Norm" (sozialer Faktor) und die „wahrgenommene Verhaltenskontrolle" (Leichtigkeit oder Schwierigkeit der Durchführung des Verhaltens) einen Einfluss auf die Absicht und nachfolgend auf das Verhalten haben.

Die Komponente „Einstellung gegenüber einem Verhalten" umfasst die verhaltensbezogene Einstellung des Pflegepersonals zu PflegeheimbewohnerInnen mit Demenz. Diese Einstellung kann positiv oder negativ ausgeprägt sein.

Die „subjektive Norm" beinhaltet die soziale Komponente. Dabei wird angenommen, dass Einstellungen und Werte der ArbeitskollegInnen, der Führungskräfte und der Gesellschaft einen Einfluss auf das eigene Verhalten haben.

Bei der dritten Komponente der „wahrgenommenen Verhaltenskontrolle" wird die Pflege von BewohnerInnen mit Demenz als leicht oder schwer empfunden. Es ist anzunehmen, dass Erfahrungen und Wissen eine wichtige Rolle spielen.

Dabei kann festgehalten werden, dass die Einstellung gegenüber einem Verhalten und die wahrgenommene Verhaltenskontrolle sich gegenseitig beeinflussen. Haben Pflegepersonen ausreichend Wissen über Demenz, ist die Einstellung eher positiv gegenüber BewohnerInnen mit Demenz.

Alle diese drei Komponenten können einen Einfluss auf die Absicht und nachfolgend auf das Verhalten nehmen. Die Absicht kann im Pflegebereich möglicherweise von Wissen, Ausbildung, Pflegebereitschaft und Berufserfahrung beeinflusst werden. Daraus folgt eine Intention, die angemessene bzw. unangemessene Pflege nach sich ziehen kann. Die Absicht der Pflegeperson beeinflusst ihr Verhalten gegenüber der BewohnerInnen.

Pflegepersonen, die eine positive Einstellung gegenüber BewohnerInnen mit Demenz sowie über ein positives Arbeitsklima, ausreichendes Wissen und Erfahrung verfügen, werden vermutlich eher die Intention haben eine angemessene Pflege durchzuführen. Dieses Pflegeverhalten wirkt sich sowohl positiv auf die Pflegepersonen als auch auf die BewohnerInnen aus.

Hingegen kann eine negative Einstellung gegenüber BewohnerInnen mit Demenz und unzureichendes Wissen zu der Intention führen, dass eher eine unangemessene Pflege durchgeführt wird. Diese Intention kann dann dazu führen, dass das Verhalten sowohl für BewohnerInnen mit Demenz als auch für das Pflegepersonal negativ ist.

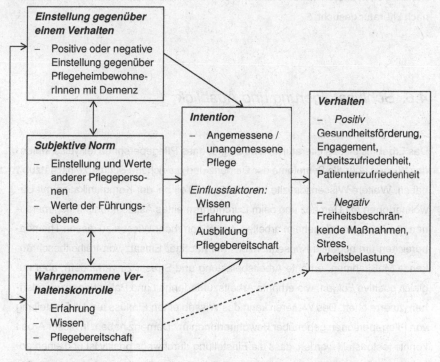

Abbildung 5: Theoretischer Bezugsrahmen in Anlehnung der Theorie von Ajzen (1991)

4.5. Limitationen und Stärken

Eine Limitation dieser Arbeit ist es, dass es sich hierbei um kein systematisches Review handelt. Die Studien wurden nur von einer Person einer Bewertung unterzogen. Das Ergebnis der Studie von Chang et al. (2010) zur Pflegebereitschaft war nicht aussagekräftig. Die Studie wurde trotz alldem hinzugezogen um aufzuzeigen, dass es zu diesem Thema sehr wenige Studien gibt. Die Stärken dieser Arbeit sind, dass eine internationale Literaturrecherche in sechs Datenbanken durchgeführt wurde. Des Weiteren wurde sowohl in englischer als auch in deutscher Sprache nach Literatur gesucht.

4.6. Schlussfolgerung und Ausblick

Das Ergebnis dieses Literaturreviews zeigte, dass Pflegepersonen teilweise fehlendes Wissen über die Symptome der Demenz und die richtige Schmerzeinschätzung haben. Weitere Wissensdefizite bestehen zum Teil bei der Kommunikation mit BewohnerInnen mit Demenz und beim Durchführen eines Assessments. Pflegepersonen, die in einem Pflegeheim arbeiten, benötigen mehr Wissen zu diesen Themenbereichen um negative Konsequenzen, wie häufiger Einsatz von freiheitbeschränkende Maßnahmen, erhöhte Arbeitsbelastung und Stress, zu verhindern, aber zugleich positive Folgen, wie erhöhte Arbeitszufriedenheit und PatientInnenzufriedenheit ‚zu erreichen. Des Weiteren kann das Wissen einen Einfluss auf die Einstellung von Pflegepersonen gegenüber BewohnerInnen mit Demenz haben. In dieser Arbeit konnte festgestellt werden, dass die Einstellung durchwegs positiv ist und einen positiven Einfluss auf Lebensqualität und PatientInnenzufriedenheit haben kann. Die Pflegebereitschaft von Pflegepersonen zu BewohnerInnen mit Demenz, wird in der Literatur hingegen kaum beschrieben.

Empfehlung für weitere Forschung

Es wäre von Interesse, das Wissen, die Einstellung und die Pflegebereitschaft von Pflegepersonen gegenüber BewohnerInnen mit Demenz in österreichischen Pflegeheimen zu erheben. Derzeit gibt es dazu noch keine Studien in Österreich. Eine Empfehlung für weitere Studien wäre, sowohl Wissen als auch Einstellung von Pflegepersonen über Demenz zu erheben. Dabei sollte evaluiert werden, inwieweit sie sich gegenseitig beeinflussen. Des Weiteren sollten die Ergebnisse getrennt nach Ausbildungsniveau dargestellt werden, um Unterschiede festmachen zu können. Im Bereich der Schmerzeinschätzung wäre eine weitere Überarbeitung der bereits vorhandenen non-verbalen Schmerzassessmentinstrumente notwendig, um sie in der Praxis einsetzen zu können.

Die Pflegebereitschaft, von Pflegepersonen zu BewohnerInnen mit Demenz, wird in der Literatur kaum beschrieben. Für weitere Studien wird nahegelegt, die Pflegebereitschaft zu erheben. Dabei sollten unterschiedliche Kontrollvariablen miterhoben werden (u.a. Wissen, Einstellung, Arbeitszufriedenheit, Arbeitsbelastung).

Empfehlung für die Praxis

Für Pflegepersonen, die mit PflegeheimbewohnerInnen mit Demenz arbeiten, sind Schulungsprogramme sinnvoll. Diese Schulungsprogramme sollten die Symptome einer Demenz, Schmerzeinschätzung, Kommunikation mit BewohnerInnen mit Demenz und Durchführen von Assessments umfassen. Das Schulungsprogramm sollte so aufgebaut werden, dass es theoretische Einheiten als auch praxisbezogene Lerneinheiten umfasst. Es ist wichtig, dass regelmäßige Auffrischungskurse angeboten werden, um fachspezifisches Wissen zu aktualisieren und weiter zu vertiefen.

Ein weiterer wichtiger Teil für die Praxis ist, dass Assessmentinstrumente vermehrt in der Praxis zur Anwendung kommen und Pflegepersonen dafür geschult werden. Der Schmerz kann bei BewohnerInnen mit Demenz, die sich verbal mitteilen können, mittels Assessmentinstrumente gut erhoben werden. Dazu geeignet wären Schmerzbewertungsskalen wie z.B. Visuelle Analogskala, Numerische Rating Skala, Gesichter-Schmerzskala (McAuliffe et al., 2012; Achterberg et al., 2013).

Bei BewohnerInnen mit Demenz, die sich nicht mehr verbal mitteilen können, wäre ein non-verbales Schmerzassessmentinstrument angebracht. Allerdings kann derzeit für kein Assessmentinstrument eine Empfehlung abgegeben werden. Es sollte jedoch bedacht werden, dass Veränderungen von Gesichtsausdruck, Verbalisierungen und Lauten, Körperbewegungen, Veränderung der zwischenmenschlichen Interaktion, der Alltagsroutine sowie des psychischen Zustandes auf einen Schmerz hindeuten können (AGS, 2002).

Für eine verbesserte Kommunikation kann der „Helpsheet" von Alzheimer's Australia (2012) für die tägliche Praxis genutzt werden. Dieser „Helpsheet" fasst kurz die wichtigsten Punkte für die richtige Kommunikation mit Personen mit Demenz zusammen. Er beschreibt welche Veränderungen bei der Kommunikation entstehen und was bei der Kommunikation mit Personen mit Demenz vermieden werden soll.

Von der Alzheimer's Association (2007 & 2009) wurden evidenzbasierte Empfehlungen veröffentlicht um besser auf die Bedürfnisse von BewohnerInnen mit Demenz eingehen zu können. Dabei werden die stadienspezifischen Symptome der Demenz und dazugehörig pflegerelevante Empfehlungen ausgesprochen. Es werden mögliche Pflegeziele formuliert und das Erheben von Symptomen beschrieben.

5. Literaturverzeichnis

Achterberg, WP, Pieper, MJC, van Dalen-Kok, AH, de Waal, MVM, Husebo, BS, Lautenbacher, S, Kunz, M, Scherder, EJA & Corbett, A 2013, 'Pain management in patients with dementia', *Clinical Interventions in Aging*, vol. 13, no. 8, pp. 1471–1482.

ADI (Alzheimer's Disease International) 2009, *World Alzheimer Report 2009*, Alzheimer's Disease International, London.

ADI (Alzheimer's Disease International) 2013, *World Alzheimer Report 2013. Journey of Caring. An analysis of long-term care for dementia*, Alzheimer's Disease International, London.

ADI (Alzheimer's Disease International) 2014, *About dementia,* Alzheimer's Disease International, London, besucht am 10.11.2014, <http://www.alz.co.uk/>.

AGS (American Geriatrics Society) Panel on Persistent Pain in Older Persons 2002, 'The management of persistent pain in older persons', *Journal of the American Geriatrics Society*, vol. 50, no. S6, pp. 205-224.

Ajzen, I 1991, 'The theory of planned behavior', *Organizational Behavior and Human Decision Processes*, vol. 50, pp. 179-211.

Alzheimer's Association 2007, *Dementia Care Practice Recommendations for Assisted Living Residences and Nursing Homes – Phase 3 End-of-Life Care*, Alzheimer's Association, Chicago.

Alzheimer's Association 2009, *Dementia Care Practice Recommendations for Assisted Living Residences and Nursing Homes – Phases 1 and 2*, Alzheimer's Association, Chicago.

Alzheimer's Association 2014, 'Alzheimer's Disease Facts and Figures', *Alzheimer's & Dementia*, vol. 10, no. 2.

Alzheimer's Australia 2011, *Pain and Dementia*, Alzheimer's Australia, Canberra, Australia, besucht am: 15.03.2015, <https://fightdementia.org.au/sites/default/files/helpsheets/Helpsheet-DementiaQandA16-PainAndDementia_english.pdf>.

Alzheimer's Australia 2012, *Communication*, Alzheimer's Australia, Canberra, Australia, besucht am: 20. 07. 2015, <https://fightdementia.org.au/sites/default/files/helpsheets/Helpsheet-CaringForSomeone01-Communication_english.pdf>.

Alzheimer's Australia 2015, *Managing Changes and in Communication*, Alzheimer's Australia, Canberra, Australia, besucht am: 15. Mai 2015, <https://fightdementia.org.au/support-and-services/i-care-for-someone-with-dementia/managing-changes-in-communication>.

Ballard, CG, Margallo-Lana, M, Fossey, J, Reichelt, K, Myint, P, Potkins, D & O'Brien, J 2001, 'A 1-year follow-up study of behavioral and psychological symptoms in dementia among people in care environments', *Journal of Clinical Psychiatry*, vol. 62, no. 8, pp. 631-636.

Bartholomeyczik, S, Linhart, S, Mayer, H & Mayer, H 2008, *Lexikon der Pflegeforschung. Begriff aus Forschung und Theorie*, Urban & Fischer, München.

Brenner, P 1994, *Stufen zur Pflegekompetenz: From Novice to Expert,* Hans Huber Verlag, Bern.

Brodaty, H, Draper, B & Low, L-F 2003, 'Nursing home staff attitudes towards residents with dementia: strain and satisfaction with work', *Journal of Advanced Nursing*, vol. 44, no. 6, pp. 583-590.

Bundesministerium für Gesundheit 2006, *Rahmenempfehlungen zum Umgang mit herausforderndem Verhalten bei Menschen mit Demenz in der stationären Altenhilfe,* Bundesministerium für Gesundheit, Witten, besucht am 16.12.2013,

<https://www.bundesgesundheitsministerium.de/fileadmin/fa_redaktion_bak/pdf_publikationen/Forschungsbericht_Rahmenempfehlungen_Umgang_Demenz.pdf>.

Bundesministerium für Gesundheit 2010, *Arbeitshilfe für die Pflegedokumentation 2010,* Bundesministerium für Gesundheit, Wien.

Bundesministerium für Gesundheit 2014, *Vaskuläre Demenz*, Bundesministerium für Gesundheit, Wien, besucht am 30.03.2015, <https://www.gesundheit.gv.at/Portal.Node/ghp/public/content/demenz-vaskulaer.html>.

Chang, E, Daly, J, Johnson, A, Harrison, K, Easterbrook, S, Bidewell, J, Stewart, H, Noel, M & Hancock, K 2009, 'Challenges for professional care of advanced dementia', *International Journal of Nursing Practice*, vol. 15, no. 1, pp. 41-47.

Chang, CH, Lin, YH, Yeh, SH & Lin, LW 2010, 'Managing problem behaviors in cognitively impaired older people: the competence and preparedness of healthcare providers in long-term care facilities', *Journal of Nursing Research*, vol 18, no. 3, pp. 164-173.

Corbett, A, Husebo, BS, Achterberg, WP, Aarsland, D, Erdal, A & Flo, E 2014, 'The importance of pain management in older people with dementia', *British Medical Bulletin*, vol. 111, no. 1, pp. 139–148.

Deutsche Gesellschaft für Allgemeinmedizin und Familienmedizin 2008, *DEGAM -Leitlinie Nr. 12: Demenz*, Deutsche Gesellschaft für Allgemeinmedizin und Familienmedizin, Düsseldorf, besucht am 06.04.2015, <http://www.degam.de/files/Inhalte/Leitlinien-Inhalte/Dokumente/DEGAM-S3-Leitlinien/LL-12_Langfassung_TJ_03_korr_01.pdf>.

Deutsches Institut für Medizinische Dokumentation und Information (DIMDI) 2014, *ICD-10-GM 2014 Systematisches Verzeichnis. Internationale statistische Klassifi-*

kation der Krankheiten und verwandter Gesundheitsprobleme. 10. Revision – German Modification, Deutsches Institut für Medizinische Dokumentation und Information, Köln.

Dijkstra, A, Buist, G & Dassen, T 1998, 'Operationalization oft he concept of 'nursing care dependency' for use in long-term care facilities', *Australian and New Zealand Journal of Mental Health Nursing*, no. 7, pp. 142-151.

Duden 2013, *Fremdwörter: Ein Nachschlagewerk für den täglichen Gebrauch*, 7th edn., Bibliographisches Institut & F.A. Brockhaus AG, Mannheim.

Eckstein, P 2014, *Repetitorium Statistik: Deskriptive Statistik - Stochastik - Induktive Statistik*, 8th edn., Springer-Gabler Verlag, Wiesbaden.

Edvardsson, D, Sandman, PO, Nay, R & Karlsson, S 2008, 'Associations between the working characteristics of nursing staff and the prevalence of behavioral symptoms in people with dementia in residential care', *International Psychogeriatrics*, vol. 20, no. 4, pp. 764-776.

Edvardsson, D, Sandman, PO, Nay, R & Karlsson, S 2009, 'Predictors of job strain in residential dementia care nursing staff', *Journal of Nursing Management*, vol. 1, no. 17, pp. 59–65.

Eurostat 2015, *Bevölkerungsstruktur und Bevölkerungsalterung*, Eurostat, European Union, besucht am 30.03.2015, <http://ec.europa.eu/eurostat/statistics-explained/index.php/Population_structure_and_ageing/de>.

Fauth, EB & Gibbons, A 2014, 'Which behavioral and psychological symptoms of dementia are the most problematic? Variability by prevalence, intensity, distress ratings, and associations with caregiver depressive symptoms', *International Journal of Geriatric Psychiatry,* vol. 29, no. 3, pp. 263-271.

Featherstone, K, James, IA, Milne, D & Maddison, C 2004, 'A controlled evaluation of a training course for staff who work with people with dementia', *Dementia*, vol. 3, no. 2, pp. 181-194.

Furåker, C & Nilsson, A 2009, 'The competence of certified nurse assistants caring for persons with dementia diseases in residential facilities', *Journal of Psychiatric and Mental Health Nursing*, vol. 16, no. 2, pp. 146-152.

Gesundheit Österreich GmbH 2013, *Alten- und Langzeitversorgung*, Gesundheit Österreich GmbH, Wien, aufgerufen am 15.12.2013, <http://www.goeg.at/de/Bereich/Alten-und-Langzeitversorgung.html>.

Gould, E & Reed, P 2009, 'Alzheimer's Association Quality Care Compaign and professional training initatives: improving hand-on are for people with dementia in the U.S.A.', *International Psychogeriatrics*, vol. 21, pp. 25-33.

Grillenberger, I & Rossa, M 2009, *Erster Österreichischer Demenzbericht. Teil 2: Gesundheitsökonomische Aspekte der Demenz*, Wiener Gebietskrankenkasse, Wien.

Grunst, S & Sure, U 2010, *Pflege konkret. Neurologie Psychiatrie*, 4th edn., Elsevier GmbH, München.

Hasson, H & Arnetz, JE 2008, 'Nursing staff competence, work strain, stress and satisfaction in elderly care: comparison of home-based care and nursing homes', *Journal of Clinical Nursing*, vol. 17, no. 4, pp. 468-481.

Herr, K, Bjoro, K & Decker, S 2006, 'Tools for assessment of pain in nonverbal older adults with dementia: a state-of-the-science review', *Journal of Pain and Symptom Management*, vol. 31, no. 2, pp. 170-92.

Herr, K, Coyne, PJ, McCaffery, M & Merkel, S 2011, 'Pain assessment in the patient unable to self-report: position statement with clinical practice recommendations', *Pain Management Nursing*, vol. 12, no. 4, pp. 230-250.

Hobday, JV, Savik, K, Smith, S & Gaugler, JE 2010, 'Feasibility of Internet Training for Care Staff of Residents with Dementia: The CARES® Program', *Journal of Gerontological Nursing*, vol. 36, no. 4, pp. 13-21.

Höwler, E 2008, *Herausforderndes Verhalten bei Menschen mit Demenz. Erleben und Strategien Pflegender*, Kohlhammer-Verlag, Stuttgart.

Hsu, MC, Moyle, W, Creedy, D & Venturato, L 2005, 'An investigation of aged care mental health knowledge of Queensland aged care nurses', *International Journal of Mental Health Nursing*, vol. 14, pp. 16–23.

Hughes, J, Bagley, H, Reilly, S, Burns, A & Challis, D 2008, 'Care staff working with people with dementia: training, knowledge and confidence', *Dementia*, vol. 7, no. 2, pp. 227-238.

Kada, S, Nygaar, HA, Mukesh, BN & Geitung, JT 2009, 'Staff attitudes towards institutionalised dementia residents', *Journal of Clinical Nursing*, vol. 18, no. 16, pp. 2383-2392.

Lee, J, Hui, E, Kng, C & Auyeung, TW 2013, 'Attitudes of long-term care staff toward dementia and their related factor', *International Psychogeratrics*, vol. 25, no.1, pp. 140-147.

KMK (Kultusministerkonferenz) 2011, *Handreichung für die Erarbeitung von Rahmenlehrplänen der Kultusministerkonferenz für den berufsbezogenen Unterricht in der Berufsschule und ihre Abstimmung mit Ausbildungsordnungen des Bundes für anerkannte Ausbildungsberufe*, Sekretariat der Kultusministerkonferenz, Berlin.

Lichtner, V, Dowding, D, Esterhuizen, P, Closs, SJ, Long, AF, Corbett, A & Briggs, M 2014, 'Pain assessment for people with dementia: a systematic review of systematic reviews of pain assessment tools', *BMC Geriatrics*, vol. 14, no. 138, pp.1-19.

Macdonald, AJD & Woods, RT 2005, 'Attitudes to dementia and dementia care held by nursing staff in U.K. "non-EMI" care homes: what difference do they make?', *International Psychogeriatrics*, vol. 17, no. 3, pp. 383-391.

Machi, LA & McEvoy, BT 2012, *The literature review. Six steps to success*, 2nd edn., Corwin, California.

Mamerow, R 2006, *Praxisanleitung in der Pflege*, Springer Verlag, Heidelberg.

Marin, B, Leichsenring, K, Rodrigues, R & Huber, M 2009, 'Who Cares? Care coordination and cooperation to enhance quality in elderly care in the European Union', *Discussion Paper for the Conference on Healthy and Dignified Ageing, Stockholm, 15-16 September 2009*, European Centre for Social Welfare Policy and Research, Wien.

Martens, JU 2009; *Einstellungen erkennen, beeinflussen und nachhaltig verändern und nachhaltig verändern. Von der Kunst das Leben aktiv zu gestalten*, Kohlhammer Verlag, Stuttgart.

McAuliffe, L, Brown, D & Fetherstonhaugh, D 2012 ,Pain and dementia: an overview of the literature', *International Journal of Older People Nursing*, vol. 7, no.3, pp. 219–226.

Pellfolk, TJ, Gustafson, Y, Bucht, G & Karlsson, S 2010, 'Effects of a Restraint Minimization Program on Staff Knowledge, Attitudes, and Practice: A Cluster Randomized Trial', *Journal oft he American Geriatrics Society*, vol. 58, no. 1, pp. 62-69.

Polit, DF & Beck, CT 2012, *Nursing Research*: *Generating and Assessing Evidence for Nursing Practice*, 9th edn., Lippincott Williams & Wilkins, Philadelphia.

Prince, M, Bryce, R, Albanese, E, Wimo, A, Ribeiro, W & Ferri, CP 2013, 'The global prevalence of dementia: A systematic review and metaanalysis', *Alzheimer's & Dementia*, vol. 9, no. 2, pp. 63-75.

Richardson, B, Kitchen, G & Livingston, G 2002, 'The effect of education on knowledge and management of elder abuse: a randomized controlled trial', *Age Ageing*, vol. 31, no. 5, pp. 335-41.

Robert-Koch-Institut 2009, *Gesundheit und Krankheit im Alter,* Robert-Koch-Institut, Berlin.

Robinson, A, Eccleston, C, Annear, M, Elliott, KE, Andrews, S, Stirling, C, Ashby, M, Donohue, C, Banks, S, Toye, C & McInerney, F 2014, 'Who Knows, Who Cares? Dementia knowledgge among nurses, care workers, and family members of people living with dementia', *Journal of Palliative Care*, vol. 30, no. 3, pp. 158-165.

Schmidt, R, Marksteiner, J, Dal Bianco, P, Ransmayr, G, Bancher, C, Benke, T, Wancata, J, Fischer, P, Leblhuber, CF, Psota, G, Ackerl, M, Alf, C, Berek, K, Croy, A, Delazer, M, Fasching, P, Frühwald, T, Fruhwürth, G, Fuchs-Nieder, B, Gatterer, G, Grossmann, J, Hinterhuber, H, Iglseder, B, Imarhiagbe, D, Jagsch, C, Jellinger, K, Kalousek, M, Kapeller, P, Ladurner, G, Lampl, C, Lechner, A, Lingg, A, Nakajima, T, Rainer, M, Reisecker, F, Spatt, J, Walch, T, Uranüs, M & Walter, A 2010, 'Konsensusstatement „Demenz 2010" der Österreichischen Alzheimer Gesellschaft', *Neuropsychiatrie*, vol. 24, no. 2, pp. 67-87.

Schüssler, S, Dassen, T & Lohrmann, C 2014, 'Prevalence of Care Dependency and Nursing Care Problems in Nursing Home Residents with Dementia: A Literature Review', *International Journal of Caring Sciences*, vol. 7, no. 2, pp. 338-352.

Schüssler, S, Dassen, T & Lohrmann, C 2015, 'Comparison of care dependency and related nursing care problems between Austrian nursing home residents with and without dementia', *European Geriatric Medicine*, vol. 6, no. 1, pp. 46-52.

Sheehan, B 2012, 'Assessment scales in dementia', *Therapeutic Advances in Neurological Disorders*, vol. 5, no. 6, pp. 349-358.

Sormunen, S, Topo, P, Eloniemi-Sulkava U, Räikkönen, O & Sarvimäki, A 2007, 'Inappropriate treatment of people with dementia in residential and day care', *Aging and mental health*, vol. 11, no. 3, pp. 246-55.

Sprangers, S, Dijkstra, K & Romijn-Luijten, A 2015, 'Communication skills training in a nursing home: effects of a brief intervention on residents and nursing aides', *Clinical Interventions in Aging*, vol. 10, pp. 311-319.

Statistik Austria 2015, *Bevölkerungsprognosen*, Statistik Austria, Wien, besucht am 06. 04. 2015, <http://www.statistik.at/web_de/statistiken/bevoelkerung/demographische_prognosen/bevoelkerungsprognosen/index.html#index1>.

Travers, CM, Beattie, E, Martin-Khan, M, Fielding, E 2013, 'A survey of the Queensland healthcare workforce: attitudes towards dementia care and training', *BMC Geriatrics*, vol. 13, no. 101, pp. 1-7.

United Nations 2013, *World Population Prospects. The 2012 Revision. Volume II: Demographic Profiles*, United Nations, New York.

Vasse, E, Vernooij-Dassen, M, Spijker, A, Rikkert, MO & Raymond, K 2010, 'A systematic review of communication strategies for people with dementia in residential and nursing homes', *International Psychogeriatrics,* vol. 22, no. 2, pp. 189–200.

WHO 2006, *Neurological Disorders: Public Health Challenges*, WHO, Schweiz.

WHO 2012, *Dementia: a public health priority*, WHO, Schweiz.

Wimo, A, Jönsson, L, Gustavsson, A, McDaid, D, Ersek, K, Georges, J, Gula`csi, L, Karpati, K, Kenigsberg, P & Valtonen, H 2010, 'The economic impact of dementia in Europe in 2008—cost estimates from the Eurocode project', *International Journal of Geriatric Psychiatry,* vol. 26, no. 8, S. 825-832.

Zimmerman, S, Williams, CS, Reed, PS, Boustani, M, Preiser, JS, Heck, E & Sloane, PD 2005a, 'Attitudes, stress and satisfaction of staff who care for residents with dementia', *The Gerontologist*, vol. 45 (Special Issue), no. 1, pp. 96-105.

Zimmerman, S, Sloane, D, Williams, CS, Reed, PS, Preisser, JS, Eckert, JK, Boustani, M & Dobbs, D 2005b, 'Dementia Care and Quality of Life in Assisted Living and Nursing Homes', *The Gerontologist*, vol. 45, no.1, pp. 133–146.

Zimmerman, S, Mitchell, M, Reed, D, Preisser, JS, Fletcher, S, Beeber, AS, Reed, P, Gould, E, Hughes, S, McConell, ES, Corazzini, KN, Lekan, D & Sloane, PD 2010, 'Outcomes of a Dementia Care Training Program for Staff in Nursing Homes and Residential Care/Assisted Living Settings', *Alzheimer's Care Today*, vol. 11, no. 2, pp. 83-99.

Zwakhalen, SM, Hamers, JP, Abu-Saad, HH & Berger, MP 2006, 'Pain in elderly people with severe dementia: a systematic review of behavioural pain assessment tools', *BMC Geriatrics*, vol. 6, no. 3, pp. 1-15.

6. Anhang 1: Suchprotokolle der Literaturrecherche

PubMed

<u>Limitationen:</u> Field: Title/Abstract / Filters: published in the last 10 years / language: english, german

Nr.	Keywords	Results
#1	"Dementia" [Mesh] OR dement* OR alzheimer* OR (cognitive* AND impair*)	37287
#2	"Residential Facilities" [Mesh] OR "Long-Term Care" [Mesh] OR long-term care OR nursing home* OR residential	15789
#3	"Nurses" [Mesh] OR "Nurses' Aides" [Mesh] OR "Nursing Staff" [Mesh] OR nurs*	36563
#4	"Knowledge" [Mesh] OR „Professional Competence" [Mesh] OR know* OR competen* OR abilit* OR aware* OR expert* OR skill*	385500
#5	**#1 AND #2 AND #3 AND #4**	**252**
#6	"Attitude" [Mesh] OR attitude* OR belief* OR convic* OR opinion* OR perspective* OR position* OR view* OR think*	176951
#7	**#1 AND #2 AND #3 AND #6**	**128**
#8	"Motivation" [Mesh] OR „Job Satisfaction" [Mesh] OR motivat* OR will* OR read* OR engagement OR satisf*	230896
#9	**#1 AND #3 AND #3 AND #8**	**151**

Cinahl

<u>Limitationen:</u> Sprache: deutsch/englisch / Date: 2004 bis 2014 / Research article

Nr.	Keywords	Results
#1	(MH "Dementia") OR dement* OR alzheimer* OR (cognitive* AND immpair*)	2801
#2	(MH"Nurse") OR (MH „Nursing Assistants") OR nurs*	14931
#3	(MH "Residential Facilities+") OR long-term care OR nursing home* OR residential	2961
#4	(MH "Knowledge+") OR (MH "Professional Competence+*") OR know* OR competen* OR abilit* OR aware* OR expert* OR skill*	29198
#5	**#1 AND #2 AND #3 AND #4**	**108**

#6	(MH "Attitude+") OR attitude* OR belief* OR convic* OR opinion* OR perspective* OR position* OR view* OR think*	49841
#7	**#1 AND #2 AND #3 AND #6**	**95**
#8	(MH "Motivation+" OR (MM "Job Satisfaction") OR motivat* OR will* OR read* OR engagement OR satisf*	20885
#9	**#1 AND #2 AND #3 AND #8**	**69**

Embase via Ovid

<u>Limitationen</u>: Publikation: 2004-2014 / Sprache: deutsch/englisch / Title/Abstract / human / article / journal review

Nr.	Keywords	Results
#1	dementia (Subject Heading exp.) OR dement* OR alzheimer* OR (cognitive* and impair*)	62238
#2	residential home (Subject heading exp.) OR long-term care OR nursing home* OR residential	39130
#3	nurse (Subject heading exp.) OR nursing assistant (Subject heading exp) OR nurs*	51075
#4	knowledge (Subject Heading exp.) OR professional competence (Subject heading exp.) OR know* OR compten* OR abilit* OR aware* OR expert* OR skill*	403937
#5	**#1 AND #2 AND #3 AND #4**	**307**
#6	attitude (Subject heading exp.) OR attitude* OR belief* OR convic* OR opinion* OR perspective*OR position* OR view* OR think*	173616
#7	**#1 AND #2 AND #3 AND #6**	**198**
#8	Motivation (Subject heading exp.) OR job satisfaction (Subject heading exp.) OR motivat* OR will* OR read* OR engagement OR satisf*	326282
#9	**#1 AND #2 AND #3 AND #8**	**306**

Cochrane via Ovid

<u>Limitationen:</u> last 10 years / Suchfeld: Titel+Abstract

Nr.	Keywords	Results
#1	Dement* OR alzheimer* OR (cognitive* AND impair*)	74
#2	Long-term care OR nursing home* OR residential	22
#3	*nurs*	154
#4	know* OR competen* OR abilit* OR aware* OR expert* OR skill*	581
#5	#1 AND #2 AND #3 AND #4	1
#6	Attitude* OR belief* OR convic* OR opinion* OR perspective* OR position* OR view* OR think*	127
#7	#1 AND #2 AND #3 AND #6	0
#8	Motivat* OR will* OR read* OR engagement OR satisf*	545
#9	#1 AND #2 AND #3 AND #8	1

Gerollt (Deutsch)

<u>Limitationen:</u> 2004-2014

Nr.	Keywords	Results
#1	Demenz* ODER Alzheimer*	1092
#2	Pflegeheim* Oder Langzeitpflege*	443
#3	Pflege* ODER Kranken*	3621
#4	Wissen ODER Fähigkeit* ODER Können	11
#5	#1 AND #2 AND #3 AND #4	0
#6	Einstellung* Oder Sichtweise*	304
#7	#1 AND #2 AND #3 AND #6	0
#8	Bereitschaft* ODER Motivation*	169
#9	#1 AND #2 AND #3 AND #8	0

Gerolit (Englisch)

Nr.	Keywords	Results
#1	Dement* ODER alzheimer*	540
#2	Nursing home* ODER long term care ODER residential	254
#3	Nurs*	202
#4	Know* ODER Skill* ODER competen*	100
#5	**#1 AND #2 AND #3 AND #4**	**3**
#6	Attitude* ODER view*	78
#7	**#1 AND #2 AND #3 AND #6**	**1**
#8	Motivation* ODER readiness	175
#9	**#1 AND #2 AND #3 AND #8**	**0**

PsychInfo

<u>Limitationen:</u> Sprache: deutsch/englisch / Journal / peer-reviewed journal / non-peer-reviewed journal / peer-reviewed status unknown, last 10 years.

Nr.	Keywords	Results
#1	dementia (Subject Heading exp.) OR dement* OR alzheimer* OR (cognitive* and impair*)	82900
#2	Nurse (Subject heading exp.) OR nurs*	60639
#3	Residential Care Institution (Subject heading exp.) OR long-term care OR nursing home* OR residential	44273
#4	Knowledge (Subject Heading exp.) OR professional competence (Subject Heading exp.) OR know* OR competen* OR abilit* OR a-ware* OR expert* OR skill*	656220
#5	**#1 AND #2 AND #3 AND #4**	**380**
#6	Attitude (Subject Heading exp.) OR attitude* OR belief* OR convic* OR opinion* OR perspective*OR position* OR view* OR think*	775295
#7	**#1 AND #2 AND #3 AND #6**	**213**
#8	Motivation (Subject Heading exp.) OR job satisfaction (Subject Heading exp.) OR motivat* OR will* OR need* OR engagement OR satisf*	590003
#9	**#1 AND #2 AND #3 AND #8**	**264**

7. Anhang 2: Bewertung der quantitativen Studien

Chang et al., 2010

Title	
Is the title a good one, succinctly suggesting key variables and the study population?	Ja (p.164)

Abstract	
Does the abstract clearly and concisely summarize the main features of the report (problem, methods, results, conclusion)?	Ja (p.164)

Introduction	
Statement of the problem o Is the problem stated unambiguously, and is it easy to identify? o Does the problem statement build a cogent, persuasive argument for the new study? o Does the problem have significance for nursing? o Is there a good match between the research problem and the paradigm and methods used? Is a quantitative approach appropriate?	Ja (p.164ff)
Hypotheses or research question o Are research questions and/or hypotheses explicitly stated? If not, is their absence justified? o Are questions and hypotheses appropriately words, with clear specification of key variables and the study population? o Are the question/hypotheses consistent with the literature review and the conceptual framework? Anmerkung: Keine Forschungsfrage oder Hypothese formuliert, Forschungsziel vorhanden – alle Variablen vorhanden (p. 165).	Teilweise
Literature review o Is the literature review up to date and based mainly on primary sources? o Does the review provide a state-of-the-art synthesis of evidence on the problem? o Does the literature review provide a sound basis for the new study?	Ja
Conceptual/theoretical framework o Are key concepts adequately defined conceptually? o Is there a conceptual/theoretical framework rationale, and/or map, and (if so) is it appropriate? If not, is the absence of one justified?	Nein

Method	
Protection of human rights	Ja (p. 166)
o Were appropriate procedures used to safeguard the right of study partici-pants? Was the study externally reviewed by an IRB/ethics review board? o Was the study designed to minimize risks and maximize benefits to partici-pants?	
Research designs	Ja (p.166)
o Was the most rigorous possible design used, given the study purpose? o Were appropriate comparisons made to enhance interpretability of the findings? o Was the number of data collection points appropriate? o Did the design minimize biases and threats to the internal, construct, and external validity of the study (e.g. was blinding used, was attrition mini-mized)?	
Population and sample	Teilweise
o Is the population described? Is the sample described in sufficient detail? o Was the best possible sampling design used to enhance the sample's rep-resentativeness? Were sampling biases minimized? o Was the sample size adequate? Was a power analysis used to estimate sample size needs? **Anmerkung** Population ausreichend beschrieben und tabellarisch dargestellt (p.167), keine Power-Analyse	
Data collection and measurements	Teilweise
o Are the operational and conceptual definitions congruent? o Were key variables operationalized using the best possible method (e.g., interviews, observations, and so on) and with adequate justification? o Are specific instruments adequately described and were they good choices, given the study purpose, variables being studied, and the study population? o Does the report provide evidence that the data collection methods yielded data that were reliable and valid? **Anmerkung** Keine Definition von "cognitive impaired", k.A dazu, wer die Experten waren, die die Inhaltsvalidität bestimmten. Fragliche Inhaltsvalidität; verwendete Fragebögen werden beschrieben und sind lt. AutoInnen reliabel und valide (p. 166f).	
Procedures	Keine Intervention
o If there was an intervention, is it adequately described, and was it rigor-ously developed and implemented? Did most participants allocated to the intervention group actually receive it? Is there evidence of intervention fi-delity? o Were data collected in a manner that minimized bias? Were the staff who collected data appropriately trained?	

Results	
Data analysis	Ja (p. 167)
o Were analyses undertaken to address each research question or test each hypothesis? o Were appropriate statistical methods used, given the level of measurement of the variables, number of groups being compared, and assumption of the tests? o Was the most powerful analytic method used (e.g., did the analysis help to control for confounding variables)? o Were Type I and Type II errors avoided or minimized? o In intervention studies, was an intention-to-treat analysis performed? o Were problems of missing values evaluated and adequately addressed?	
Findings	Teilweise
o Is information about statistical significance presented? Is information about effect size and precision of estimates (confidence intervals) presented? o Are the finding adequately summarized, with good use of tables and figures? o Are finding reported in a manner that facilitates a meta-analysis, and with sufficient information needed for EBP? **Anmerkung:** p-Werte angeführt, Ergebnisse werden übersichtlich dargestellt, Tabellen vorhanden (p. 167ff), keine CI; Ergebnis zu Pflegebereitschaft nicht aussagekräftig.	

Discussion	
Interpretation of the findings	Teilweise
o Are all major findings interpreted and discussed within the context of prior research and/or the study's conceptual framework? o Are causal inferences, if any, justified? o Are interpretations well-founded and consistent with the study's limitations? o Does the report address the issue of the generalizability of the findings? **Anmerkung:** Keine Interpretation für das Ergebnis Pflegebereitschaft – der Grad der Ausprägung der Pflegebereitschaft geht nicht hervor. Generalisierbarkeit nicht gegeben.	(p.169f)
Implications/recommendations	Ja (p.171)
o Do the researchers discuss the implications of the study for clinical practice or further research – and are those implications reasonable and complete?	

Global Issues	
Presentation o Is the report well-written, organized, and sufficiently detailed for critical analysis? o In intervention studies, is a CONSORT flow chart provides to show the flow of participants in the study? o Is the report written in a manner that makes the findings accessible to practicing nurses?	Ja
Researcher credibility o Do the researchers' clinical, substantive, or methodologic qualifications and experience enhance confidence in the findings and their interpretation?	Ja
Summary assessment o Despite any limitations, do the study findings appear to be valid, do you have confidence in the truth value of the results? o Does the study contribute any meaningful evidence that can be used in nursing practice or that is useful to the nursing discipline?	Ja

Featherstone et al., 2004

Title	
Is the title a good one, succinctly suggesting key variables and the study population?	Ja (p.181))

Abstract	
Does the abstract clearly and concisely summarize the main features of the report (problem, methods, results, conclusion)? **Anmerkung:** Problem wird nicht beschrieben, andere Variablen vorhanden (p. 181).	Teilweise

Introduction	
Statement of the problem o Is the problem stated unambiguously, and is it easy to identify? o Does the problem statement build a cogent, persuasive argument for the new study? o Does the problem have significance for nursing? o Is there a good match between the research problem and the paradigm and methods used? Is a quantitative approach appropriate?	Ja (p.181ff)
Hypotheses or research question o Are research questions and/or hypotheses explicitly stated? If not, is their absence justified? o Are questions and hypotheses appropriately words, with clear specification of key variables and the study population? o Are the question/hypotheses consistent with the literature review and the conceptual framework?	Ja (p.187)
Literature review o Is the literature review up to date and based mainly on primary sources? o Does the review provide a state-of-the-art synthesis of evidence on the problem? o Does the literature review provide a sound basis for the new study?	Ja
Conceptual/theoretical framework o Are key concepts adequately defined conceptually? o Is there a conceptual/theoretical framework rationale, and/or map, and (if so) is it appropriate? If not, is the absence of one justified?	Nein

Method	
Protection of human rights o Were appropriate procedures used to safeguard the right of study participants? Was the study externally reviewed by an IRB/ethics review board? o Was the study designed to minimize risks and maximize benefits to participants?	Ja (p. 185)
Research designs o Was the most rigorous possible design used, given the study purpose? o Were appropriate comparisons made to enhance interpretability of the findings? o Was the number of data collection points appropriate? o Did the design minimize biases and threats to the internal, construct, and external validity of the study (e.g. was blinding used, was attrition minimized)? **Anmkerung** Auswahl der Häuser nach dem Prinzip "first come first serve" → Bias-Gefahr	Teilweise
Population and sample o Is the population described? Is the sample described in sufficient detail? o Was the best possible sampling design used to enhance the sample's representativeness? Were sampling biases minimized? o Was the sample size adequate? Was a power analysis used to estimate sample size needs? **Anmerkung** Kleine Stichprobe (wegen Pilottest), keine Beschreibung wer unter "care worker" fällt, k.A. zur Rücklaufquote, keine Power-Analyse	Teilweise
Data collection and measurements o Are the operational and conceptual definitions congruent? o Were key variables operationalized using the best possible method (e.g., interviews, observations, and so on) and with adequate justification? o Are specific instruments adequately described and were they good choices, given the study purpose, variables being studied, and the study population? o Does the report provide evidence that the data collection methods yielded data that were reliable and valid?	Ja (p. 187)
Procedures o If there was an intervention, is it adequately described, and was it rigorously developed and implemented? Did most participants allocated to the intervention group actually receive it? Is there evidence of intervention fidelity? o Were data collected in a manner that minimized bias? Were the staff who collected data appropriately trained?	Ja (p.185ff)

Results	
<u>Data analysis</u> o Were analyses undertaken to address each research question or test each hypothesis? o Were appropriate statistical methods used, given the level of measurement of the variables, number of groups being compared, and assumption of the tests? o Was the most powerful analytic method used (e.g., did the analysis help to control for confounding variables)? o Were Type I and Type II errors avoided or minimized? o In intervention studies, was an intention-to-treat analysis performed? o Were problems of missing values evaluated and adequately addressed?	Ja (p. 188)
<u>Findings</u> o Is information about statistical significance presented? Is information about effect size and precision of estimates (confidence intervals) presented? o Are the finding adequately summarized, with good use of tables and figures? o Are finding reported in a manner that facilitates a meta-analysis, and with sufficient information needed for EBP?	Ja (p.188f)

Discussion	
<u>Interpretation of the findings</u> o Are all major findings interpreted and discussed within the context of prior research and/or the study's conceptual framework? o Are causal inferences, if any, justified? o Are interpretations well-founded and consistent with the study's limitations? o Does the report address the issue of the generalizability of the findings? **Anmerkung** Ergebnisse werden interpretiert und diskutiert (p. 189ff), Generalisierbarkeit der Ergebnisse ist nicht gegeben.	Teilweise
<u>Implications/recommendations</u> o Do the researchers discuss the implications of the study for clinical practice or further research – and are those implications reasonable and complete?	Ja (p.191)

Global Issues	
Presentation o Is the report well-written, organized, and sufficiently detailed for critical analysis? o In intervention studies, is a CONSORT flow chart provides to show the flow of participants in the study? o Is the report written in a manner that makes the findings accessible to practicing nurses?	Ja
Researcher credibility o Do the researchers' clinical, substantive, or methodologic qualifications and experience enhance confidence in the findings and their interpretation?	Ja
Summary assessment o Despite any limitations, do the study findings appear to be valid, do you have confidence in the truth value of the results? o Does the study contribute any meaningful evidence that can be used in nursing practice or that is useful to the nursing discipline?	Ja

Title	
Is the title a good one, succinctly suggesting key variables and the study population?	Ja (p.25)

Abstract	
Does the abstract clearly and concisely summarize the main features of the report (problem, methods, results, conclusion)?	Ja (p.25)

Introduction	
Statement of the problem ○ Is the problem stated unambiguously, and is it easy to identify? ○ Does the problem statement build a cogent, persuasive argument for the new study? ○ Does the problem have significance for nursing? ○ Is there a good match between the research problem and the paradigm and methods used? Is a quantitative approach appropriate?	Ja (p.25f)
Hypotheses or research question ○ Are research questions and/or hypotheses explicitly stated? If not, is their absence justified? ○ Are questions and hypotheses appropriately words, with clear specification of key variables and the study population? ○ Are the question/hypotheses consistent with the literature review and the conceptual framework? **Anmerkung:** Keine Forschungsfrage oder Hypothese formuliert, Ziel der Pilotstudie wird angegeben (p. 29).	Teilweise
Literature review ○ Is the literature review up to date and based mainly on primary sources? ○ Does the review provide a state-of-the-art synthesis of evidence on the problem? ○ Does the literature review provide a sound basis for the new study?	Ja
Conceptual/theoretical framework ○ Are key concepts adequately defined conceptually? ○ Is there a conceptual/theoretical framework rationale, and/or map, and (if so) is it appropriate? If not, is the absence of one justified?	Nein

Method	
Protection of human rights o Were appropriate procedures used to safeguard the right of study partici- pants? Was the study externally reviewed by an IRB/ethics review board? o Was the study designed to minimize risks and maximize benefits to partici- pants?	Ja (p. 29)
Research designs o Was the most rigorous possible design used, given the study purpose? o Were appropriate comparisons made to enhance interpretability of the findings? o Was the number of data collection points appropriate? o Did the design minimize biases and threats to the internal, construct, and external validity of the study (e.g. was blinding used, was attrition mini- mized)?	Ja (p.29)
Population and sample o Is the population described? Is the sample described in sufficient detail? o Was the best possible sampling design used to enhance the sample's rep- resentativeness? Were sampling biases minimized? o Was the sample size adequate? Was a power analysis used to estimate sample size needs? **Anmerkung** Studienpopulation nicht ausreichend beschrieben –> keine demografischen Daten, nicht übersichtlich.	Teilweise
Data collection and measurements o Are the operational and conceptual definitions congruent? o Were key variables operationalized using the best possible method (e.g., interviews, observations, and so on) and with adequate justification? o Are specific instruments adequately described and were they good choices, given the study purpose, variables being studied, and the study population? o Does the report provide evidence that the data collection methods yielded data that were reliable and valid? **Anmerkung** Datenerhebung wird ausreichend ausreichend beschreiben (p. 29ff); ver- wendete Fragebögen werden nicht erklärt -> aber Literaturhinweis angeführt (p. 30)	Teilweise
Procedures o If there was an intervention, is it adequately described, and was it rigor- ously developed and implemented? Did most participants allocated to the intervention group actually receive it? Is there evidence of intervention fi- delity? o Were data collected in a manner that minimized bias? Were the staff who collected data appropriately trained?	Ja (p.27ff)

Results	
Data analysis	Teilweise
o Were analyses undertaken to address each research question or test each hypothesis? o Were appropriate statistical methods used, given the level of measurement of the variables, number of groups being compared, and assumption of the tests? o Was the most powerful analytic method used (e.g., did the analysis help to control for confounding variables)? o Were Type I and Type II errors avoided or minimized? o In intervention studies, was an intention-to-treat analysis performed? o Were problems of missing values evaluated and adequately addressed? **Anmerkung** Keine Beschreibung welche statistsiche Methoden zur Datenanalyse angwandt wurden.	
Findings	Ja (p.30ff)
o Is information about statistical significance presented? Is information about effect size and precision of estimates (confidence intervals) presented? o Are the finding adequately summarized, with good use of tables and figures? o Are finding reported in a manner that facilitates a meta-analysis, and with sufficient information needed for EBP?	

Discussion	
Interpretation of the findings	Nein
o Are all major findings interpreted and discussed within the context of prior research and/or the study's conceptual framework? o Are causal inferences, if any, justified? o Are interpretations well-founded and consistent with the study's limitations? o Does the report address the issue of the generalizability of the findings? **Anmerkung**: Ergebnisse wurden nicht mit anderen Studien verglichen, keine Limitation/Schwäche der Studie angeben .	
Implications/recommendations	Ja (p.33)
o Do the researchers discuss the implications of the study for clinical practice or further research – and are those implications reasonable and complete?	

Global Issues	
Presentation o Is the report well-written, organized, and sufficiently detailed for critical analysis? o In intervention studies, is a CONSORT flow chart provides to show the flow of participants in the study? o Is the report written in a manner that makes the findings accessible to practicing nurses? **Anmerkung** Der Aufbau der Studie ist unübersichtlich -- > einzelne Abschnitte sind schwer zu finden.	Teilweise
Researcher credibility o Do the researchers' clinical, substantive, or methodologic qualifications and experience enhance confidence in the findings and their interpretation?	Ja
Summary assessment o Despite any limitations, do the study findings appear to be valid, do you have confidence in the truth value of the results? o Does the study contribute any meaningful evidence that can be used in nursing practice or that is useful to the nursing discipline?	Ja

Title	
Is the title a good one, succinctly suggesting key variables and the study population?	Ja (p.468)

Abstract	
Does the abstract clearly and concisely summarize the main features of the report (problem, methods, results, conclusion)?	Ja (p.468f)

Introduction	
Statement of the problem	Ja (p.469f)
o Is the problem stated unambiguously, and is it easy to identify? o Does the problem statement build a cogent, persuasive argument for the new study? o Does the problem have significance for nursing? o Is there a good match between the research problem and the paradigm and methods used? Is a quantitative approach appropriate?	
Hypotheses or research question	Ja (p.470)
o Are research questions and/or hypotheses explicitly stated? If not, is their absence justified? o Are questions and hypotheses appropriately words, with clear specification of key variables and the study population? o Are the question/hypotheses consistent with the literature review and the conceptual framework?	
Literature review	Ja (469f)
o Is the literature review up to date and based mainly on primary sources? o Does the review provide a state-of-the-art synthesis of evidence on the problem? o Does the literature review provide a sound basis for the new study?	
Conceptual/theoretical framework	Nein
o Are key concepts adequately defined conceptually? o Is there a conceptual/theoretical framework rationale, and/or map, and (if so) is it appropriate? If not, is the absence of one justified?	

Method	
Protection of human rights	Ja (p. 473)
o Were appropriate procedures used to safeguard the right of study participants? Was the study externally reviewed by an IRB/ethics review board? o Was the study designed to minimize risks and maximize benefits to participants?	
Research designs	Ja (p.470f)
o Was the most rigorous possible design used, given the study purpose? o Were appropriate comparisons made to enhance interpretability of the findings? o Was the number of data collection points appropriate? o Did the design minimize biases and threats to the internal, construct, and external validity of the study (e.g. was blinding used, was attrition minimized)?	
Population and sample	Teilweise
o Is the population described? Is the sample described in sufficient detail? o Was the best possible sampling design used to enhance the sample's representativeness? Were sampling biases minimized? o Was the sample size adequate? Was a power analysis used to estimate sample size needs? **Anmerkung** Studienpopulation ausreichend beschrieben (p.470), Power-Analyse durchgeführt (p. 472). Rücklaufquote in beiden Pflegeheimen unterschiedlich, unterschiedliche Samplinggröße in beiden Pflegeheimen (p.473),	
Data collection and measurements	Teilweise
o Are the operational and conceptual definitions congruent? o Were key variables operationalized using the best possible method (e.g., interviews, observations, and so on) and with adequate justification? o Are specific instruments adequately described and were they good choices, given the study purpose, variables being studied, and the study population? o Does the report provide evidence that the data collection methods yielded data that were reliable and valid? **Anmerkung** Fragebögen werden ausreichend beschrieben, keine Validität der Fragebögen angeführt, Cronbach's alpha wird angeführt (p.471ff)	
Procedures	Ja (p.471)
o If there was an intervention, is it adequately described, and was it rigorously developed and implemented? Did most participants allocated to the intervention group actually receive it? Is there evidence of intervention fidelity? o Were data collected in a manner that minimized bias? Were the staff who collected data appropriately trained?	

Results	
<u>Data analysis</u> o Were analyses undertaken to address each research question or test each hypothesis? o Were appropriate statistical methods used, given the level of measurement of the variables, number of groups being compared, and assumption of the tests? o Was the most powerful analytic method used (e.g., did the analysis help to control for confounding variables)? o Were Type I and Type II errors avoided or minimized? o In intervention studies, was an intention-to-treat analysis performed? o Were problems of missing values evaluated and adequately addressed?	Ja (p.473ff)
<u>Findings</u> o Is information about statistical significance presented? Is information about effect size and precision of estimates (confidence intervals) presented? o Are the finding adequately summarized, with good use of tables and figures? o Are finding reported in a manner that facilitates a meta-analysis, and with sufficient information needed for EBP?	Ja (p.473ff)

Discussion	
<u>Interpretation of the findings</u> o Are all major findings interpreted and discussed within the context of prior research and/or the study's conceptual framework? o Are causal inferences, if any, justified? o Are interpretations well-founded and consistent with the study's limitations? o Does the report address the issue of the generalizability of the findings?	Ja (p.477ff)
<u>Implications/recommendations</u> o Do the researchers discuss the implications of the study for clinical practice or further research – and are those implications reasonable and complete?	Ja (p.479f)

Global Issues	
Presentation o Is the report well-written, organized, and sufficiently detailed for critical analysis? o In intervention studies, is a CONSORT flow chart provides to show the flow of participants in the study? o Is the report written in a manner that makes the findings accessible to practicing nurses?	Ja
Researcher credibility o Do the researchers' clinical, substantive, or methodologic qualifications and experience enhance confidence in the findings and their interpretation?	Ja
Summary assessment o Despite any limitations, do the study findings appear to be valid, do you have confidence in the truth value of the results? o Does the study contribute any meaningful evidence that can be used in nursing practice or that is useful to the nursing discipline?	Ja

Hobday et al., 2010

Title	
Is the title a good one, succinctly suggesting key variables and the study population?	Ja (p.1)

Abstract	
Does the abstract clearly and concisely summarize the main features of the report (problem, methods, results, conclusion)? **Anmerkung** Keine Problembeschreibung, anderen Variablen vorhanden (p.1)	Teilweise

Introduction	
<u>Statement of the problem</u> o Is the problem stated unambiguously, and is it easy to identify? o Does the problem statement build a cogent, persuasive argument for the new study? o Does the problem have significance for nursing? o Is there a good match between the research problem and the paradigm and methods used? Is a quantitative approach appropriate?	Ja (p.2ff)
<u>Hypotheses or research question</u> o Are research questions and/or hypotheses explicitly stated? If not, is their absence justified? o Are questions and hypotheses appropriately words, with clear specification of key variables and the study population? o Are the question/hypotheses consistent with the literature review and the conceptual framework? **Anmerkung**: Keine Forschungsfrage oder Hypothese formuliert, ausführliche Zielformulierung vorhanden (p. 2f).	Teilweise
<u>Literature review</u> o Is the literature review up to date and based mainly on primary sources? o Does the review provide a state-of-the-art synthesis of evidence on the problem? o Does the literature review provide a sound basis for the new study?	Ja
<u>Conceptual/theoretical framework</u> o Are key concepts adequately defined conceptually? o Is there a conceptual/theoretical framework rationale, and/or map, and (if so) is it appropriate? If not, is the absence of one justified?	Ja (p.3)

Method	
Protection of human rights o Were appropriate procedures used to safeguard the right of study participants? Was the study externally reviewed by an IRB/ethics review board? o Was the study designed to minimize risks and maximize benefits to participants?	Ja (p. 3)
Research designs o Was the most rigorous possible design used, given the study purpose? o Were appropriate comparisons made to enhance interpretability of the findings? o Was the number of data collection points appropriate? o Did the design minimize biases and threats to the internal, construct, and external validity of the study (e.g. was blinding used, was attrition minimized)?	Ja (p. 4)
Population and sample o Is the population described? Is the sample described in sufficient detail? o Was the best possible sampling design used to enhance the sample's representativeness? Were sampling biases minimized? o Was the sample size adequate? Was a power analysis used to estimate sample size needs? **Anmerkung** Studienpopulation ausreichend beschrieben (p.4), geringe StudienteilnehmerInnen (p. 7),	Teilweise
Data collection and measurements o Are the operational and conceptual definitions congruent? o Were key variables operationalized using the best possible method (e.g., interviews, observations, and so on) and with adequate justification? o Are specific instruments adequately described and were they good choices, given the study purpose, variables being studied, and the study population? o Does the report provide evidence that the data collection methods yielded data that were reliable and valid?	Ja (p. 4)
Procedures o If there was an intervention, is it adequately described, and was it rigorously developed and implemented? Did most participants allocated to the intervention group actually receive it? Is there evidence of intervention fidelity? o Were data collected in a manner that minimized bias? Were the staff who collected data appropriately trained?	Ja (p.3)

Results	
Data analysis o Were analyses undertaken to address each research question or test each hypothesis? o Were appropriate statistical methods used, given the level of measurement of the variables, number of groups being compared, and assumption of the tests? o Was the most powerful analytic method used (e.g., did the analysis help to control for confounding variables)? o Were Type I and Type II errors avoided or minimized? o In intervention studies, was an intention-to-treat analysis performed? o Were problems of missing values evaluated and adequately addressed?	Ja (p. 4)
Findings o Is information about statistical significance presented? Is information about effect size and precision of estimates (confidence intervals) presented? o Are the finding adequately summarized, with good use of tables and figures? o Are finding reported in a manner that facilitates a meta-analysis, and with sufficient information needed for EBP?	Ja (p. 4ff)

Discussion	
Interpretation of the findings o Are all major findings interpreted and discussed within the context of prior research and/or the study's conceptual framework? o Are causal inferences, if any, justified? o Are interpretations well-founded and consistent with the study's limitations? o Does the report address the issue of the generalizability of the findings?	Ja (p. 6f)
Implications/recommendations o Do the researchers discuss the implications of the study for clinical practice or further research – and are those implications reasonable and complete?	Ja (p.7)

Global Issues	
Presentation o Is the report well-written, organized, and sufficiently detailed for critical analysis? o In intervention studies, is a CONSORT flow chart provides to show the flow of participants in the study? o Is the report written in a manner that makes the findings accessible to practicing nurses?	Ja

Researcher credibility	Ja
o Do the researchers' clinical, substantive, or methodologic qualifications and experience enhance confidence in the findings and their interpretation?	
Summary assessment	Ja
o Despite any limitations, do the study findings appear to be valid, do you have confidence in the truth value of the results? o Does the study contribute any meaningful evidence that can be used in nursing practice or that is useful to the nursing discipline?	

Hsu et al., 2005

Title	
Is the title a good one, succinctly suggesting key variables and the study population?	Ja (p.16)

Abstract	
Does the abstract clearly and concisely summarize the main features of the report (problem, methods, results, conclusion)?	Ja (p.16)

Introduction	
Statement of the problem o Is the problem stated unambiguously, and is it easy to identify? o Does the problem statement build a cogent, persuasive argument for the new study? o Does the problem have significance for nursing? o Is there a good match between the research problem and the paradigm and methods used? Is a quantitative approach appropriate?	Ja (p.16f)
Hypotheses or research question o Are research questions and/or hypotheses explicitly stated? If not, is their absence justified? o Are questions and hypotheses appropriately words, with clear specification of key variables and the study population? o Are the question/hypotheses consistent with the literature review and the conceptual framework? **Anmerkung** Keine Forschungsfrage oder Hypothese explizit angeführt, Forschungsziel ausführlich beschreiben (p.17)	Teilweise
Literature review o Is the literature review up to date and based mainly on primary sources? o Does the review provide a state-of-the-art synthesis of evidence on the problem? o Does the literature review provide a sound basis for the new study?	Ja
Conceptual/theoretical framework o Are key concepts adequately defined conceptually? o Is there a conceptual/theoretical framework rationale, and/or map, and (if so) is it appropriate? If not, is the absence of one justified?	Nein

Method	
Protection of human rights o Were appropriate procedures used to safeguard the right of study partici-pants? Was the study externally reviewed by an IRB/ethics review board? o Was the study designed to minimize risks and maximize benefits to partici-pants?	Ja (p.17)
Research designs o Was the most rigorous possible design used, given the study purpose? o Were appropriate comparisons made to enhance interpretability of the findings? o Was the number of data collection points appropriate? o Did the design minimize biases and threats to the internal, construct, and external validity of the study (e.g. was blinding used, was attrition mini-mized)?	Ja (p.17f)
Population and sample o Is the population described? Is the sample described in sufficient detail? o Was the best possible sampling design used to enhance the sample's rep-resentativeness? Were sampling biases minimized? o Was the sample size adequate? Was a power analysis used to estimate sample size needs? **Anmerkung** Population ausreichend beschrieben (p.18), Repräsentativität lt. Autoren geg-eben (p.18), Fragebögen vom "Care Manager" der jeweiligen Einrichtung aus-geteilt (p.18) Befragte konnten möglicherweise ein Lehrbuch zur Hilfe nehmen oder andere KollegInnen befragen (p.20), keine Power-Analyse durchgeführt,	Teilweise
Data collection and measurements o Are the operational and conceptual definitions congruent? o Were key variables operationalized using the best possible method (e.g., interviews, observations, and so on) and with adequate justification? o Are specific instruments adequately described and were they good choices, given the study purpose, variables being studied, and the study population? o Does the report provide evidence that the data collection methods yielded data that were reliable and valid?	Ja (p.17f)
Procedures o If there was an intervention, is it adequately described, and was it rigor-ously developed and implemented? Did most participants allocated to the intervention group actually receive it? Is there evidence of intervention fi-delity? o Were data collected in a manner that minimized bias? Were the staff who collected data appropriately trained?	Ja (p.18)

Results	
Data analysis ○ Were analyses undertaken to address each research question or test each hypothesis? ○ Were appropriate statistical methods used, given the level of measurement of the variables, number of groups being compared, and assumption of the tests? ○ Was the most powerful analytic method used (e.g., did the analysis help to control for confounding variables)? ○ Were Type I and Type II errors avoided or minimized? ○ In intervention studies, was an intention-to-treat analysis performed? ○ Were problems of missing values evaluated and adequately addressed?	Ja (p.18f)
Findings ○ Is information about statistical significance presented? Is information about effect size and precision of estimates (confidence intervals) presented? ○ Are the finding adequately summarized, with good use of tables and figures? ○ Are finding reported in a manner that facilitates a meta-analysis, and with sufficient information needed for EBP? **Anmerkung** p-Werte werden angeführt (p.19), keine CI, Ergebnisse werden übersichtlich in Tabellen und Textform dargestellt (p.18f)	Teilweise

Discussion	
Interpretation of the findings ○ Are all major findings interpreted and discussed within the context of prior research and/or the study's conceptual framework? ○ Are causal inferences, if any, justified? ○ Are interpretations well-founded and consistent with the study's limitations? ○ Does the report address the issue of the generalizability of the findings? **Anmerkung** Ergebnisse werden mit anderer Literatur verglichen und diskutiert (p.19ff), k.A. zur Generalisierbarkeit	Teilweise
Implications/recommendations ○ Do the researchers discuss the implications of the study for clinical practice or further research – and are those implications reasonable and complete? **Anmerkung** Geringe Beschreibung über zukünftige Forschungsarbeiten (p.22)	Teilweise

Global Issues	
Presentation o Is the report well-written, organized, and sufficiently detailed for critical analysis? o In intervention studies, is a CONSORT flow chart provides to show the flow of participants in the study? o Is the report written in a manner that makes the findings accessible to practicing nurses?	Ja
Researcher credibility o Do the researchers' clinical, substantive, or methodologic qualifications and experience enhance confidence in the findings and their interpretation?	Ja
Summary assessment o Despite any limitations, do the study findings appear to be valid, do you have confidence in the truth value of the results? o Does the study contribute any meaningful evidence that can be used in nursing practice or that is useful to the nursing discipline?	Ja

Hughes et al., 2008

Title	
Is the title a good one, succinctly suggesting key variables and the study population?	Teilweise
Anmerkung: Setting nicht beschrieben, andere Variablen vorhanden (p.227)	

Abstract	
Does the abstract clearly and concisely summarize the main features of the report (problem, methods, results, conclusion)?	Ja (p.227)

Introduction	
Statement of the problem o Is the problem stated unambiguously, and is it easy to identify? o Does the problem statement build a cogent, persuasive argument for the new study? o Does the problem have significance for nursing? o Is there a good match between the research problem and the paradigm and methods used? Is a quantitative approach appropriate?	Ja (p.227f)
Hypotheses or research question o Are research questions and/or hypotheses explicitly stated? If not, is their absence justified? o Are questions and hypotheses appropriately words, with clear specification of key variables and the study population? o Are the question/hypotheses consistent with the literature review and the conceptual framework? **Anmerkung** Keine Forschungsfrage oder Hypothese explizit angeführt, Forschungsziel nicht klar erkennbar (p.229)	Nein
Literature review o Is the literature review up to date and based mainly on primary sources? o Does the review provide a state-of-the-art synthesis of evidence on the problem? o Does the literature review provide a sound basis for the new study?	Ja
Conceptual/theoretical framework o Are key concepts adequately defined conceptually? o Is there a conceptual/theoretical framework rationale, and/or map, and (if so) is it appropriate? If not, is the absence of one justified?	Nein

Method	
Protection of human rights o Were appropriate procedures used to safeguard the right of study partici-pants? Was the study externally reviewed by an IRB/ethics review board? o Was the study designed to minimize risks and maximize benefits to partici-pants? **Anmerkung** k.A. zur Ethikkommission, , Angaben vorhanden, dass Daten vertraulich behandelt werden (p.229)	Teilweise
Research designs o Was the most rigorous possible design used, given the study purpose? o Were appropriate comparisons made to enhance interpretability of the findings? o Was the number of data collection points appropriate? o Did the design minimize biases and threats to the internal, construct, and external validity of the study (e.g. was blinding used, was attrition mini-mized)?	Ja (p.229)
Population and sample o Is the population described? Is the sample described in sufficient detail? o Was the best possible sampling design used to enhance the sample's rep-resentativeness? Were sampling biases minimized? o Was the sample size adequate? Was a power analysis used to estimate sample size needs? **Anmerkung** Population wird ausreichend beschrieben (p.230), möglicher Sampling-Bias: nicht alle Pflegepersonen erreicht (p.234), keine Power-Analyse durchgeführt	Teilweise
Data collection and measurements o Are the operational and conceptual definitions congruent? o Were key variables operationalized using the best possible method (e.g., interviews, observations, and so on) and with adequate justification? o Are specific instruments adequately described and were they good choices, given the study purpose, variables being studied, and the study population? o Does the report provide evidence that the data collection methods yielded data that were reliable and valid? **Anmerkung** Keine Definition von Demenz, Fragebogen wird beschrieben (p. 230), k.A. zu psychometrische Eigenschaften	Teilweise

Procedures	Ja (p.229)
o If there was an intervention, is it adequately described, and was it rigorously developed and implemented? Did most participants allocated to the intervention group actually receive it? Is there evidence of intervention fidelity? o Were data collected in a manner that minimized bias? Were the staff who collected data appropriately trained?	

Results	
Data analysis	Ja (p.230)
o Were analyses undertaken to address each research question or test each hypothesis? o Were appropriate statistical methods used, given the level of measurement of the variables, number of groups being compared, and assumption of the tests? o Was the most powerful analytic method used (e.g., did the analysis help to control for confounding variables)? o Were Type I and Type II errors avoided or minimized? o In intervention studies, was an intention-to-treat analysis performed? o Were problems of missing values evaluated and adequately addressed?	
Findings	Teilweise
o Is information about statistical significance presented? Is information about effect size and precision of estimates (confidence intervals) presented? o Are the finding adequately summarized, with good use of tables and figures? o Are finding reported in a manner that facilitates a meta-analysis, and with sufficient information needed for EBP? **Anmerkung** Keine Trennung zwischen care/nursing staff und senior care staff, keine Trennung bei den Ergebnissen zwischen den unterschiedlichen Häusern, p-Wert angegeben (p.233), keine CI, Ergebnisse in Tabellen dargestellt (p. 231ff)	

Discussion	
Interpretation of the findings	Teilweise
o Are all major findings interpreted and discussed within the context of prior research and/or the study's conceptual framework? o Are causal inferences, if any, justified? o Are interpretations well-founded and consistent with the study's limitations? o Does the report address the issue of the generalizability of the findings? **Anmerkung** Ergebnisse werden diskutiert (p.235f), Limitationen angeführt (p.243), k.A. zur Generalisierbarkeit	

Implications/recommendations	Teilweise
o Do the researchers discuss the implications of the study for clinical practice or further research – and are those implications reasonable and complete? **Anmerkung** Nicht ausführlich beschrieben (p.236)	

Global Issues	
Presentation o Is the report well-written, organized, and sufficiently detailed for critical analysis? o In intervention studies, is a CONSORT flow chart provides to show the flow of participants in the study? o Is the report written in a manner that makes the findings accessible to practicing nurses?	Ja
Researcher credibility o Do the researchers' clinical, substantive, or methodologic qualifications and experience enhance confidence in the findings and their interpretation?	Ja
Summary assessment o Despite any limitations, do the study findings appear to be valid, do you have confidence in the truth value of the results? o Does the study contribute any meaningful evidence that can be used in nursing practice or that is useful to the nursing discipline?	Ja

Kada et al., 2009

Title	
Is the title a good one, succinctly suggesting key variables and the study population?	Ja (p.2383)

Abstract	
Does the abstract clearly and concisely summarize the main features of the report (problem, methods, results, conclusion)? **Anmerkung** Problem wird nicht beschrieben, andere Variablen vorhanden (p.2383)	Teilweise

Introduction	
<u>Statement of the problem</u> o Is the problem stated unambiguously, and is it easy to identify? o Does the problem statement build a cogent, persuasive argument for the new study? o Does the problem have significance for nursing? o Is there a good match between the research problem and the paradigm and methods used? Is a quantitative approach appropriate?	Ja (p.2383ff)
<u>Hypotheses or research question</u> o Are research questions and/or hypotheses explicitly stated? If not, is their absence justified? o Are questions and hypotheses appropriately words, with clear specification of key variables and the study population? o Are the question/hypotheses consistent with the literature review and the conceptual framework? **Anmerkung** Keine Forschungsfrage oder Hypothese explizit angeführt, Forschungsziel ausführlich beschreiben	Teilweise
<u>Literature review</u> o Is the literature review up to date and based mainly on primary sources? o Does the review provide a state-of-the-art synthesis of evidence on the problem? o Does the literature review provide a sound basis for the new study?	Ja
<u>Conceptual/theoretical framework</u> o Are key concepts adequately defined conceptually? o Is there a conceptual/theoretical framework rationale, and/or map, and (if so) is it appropriate? If not, is the absence of one justified?	Nein

Method	
Protection of human rights o Were appropriate procedures used to safeguard the right of study partici-pants? Was the study externally reviewed by an IRB/ethics review board? o Was the study designed to minimize risks and maximize benefits to partici-pants?	Ja (p.2386)
Research designs o Was the most rigorous possible design used, given the study purpose? o Were appropriate comparisons made to enhance interpretability of the findings? o Was the number of data collection points appropriate? o Did the design minimize biases and threats to the internal, construct, and external validity of the study (e.g. was blinding used, was attrition mini-mized)?	Ja (p.2385)
Population and sample o Is the population described? Is the sample described in sufficient detail? o Was the best possible sampling design used to enhance the sample's rep-resentativeness? Were sampling biases minimized? o Was the sample size adequate? Was a power analysis used to estimate sample size needs? **Anmerkung** Studienpopulation ausreichend beschrieben (p.2385f), Stationsschwester (head nurse) teilte Fragebögen aus (p.2385) – k.A. wie Fragebögen wieder eingesammelt wurden, keine Power-Analyse durchgeführt	Teilweise
Data collection and measurements o Are the operational and conceptual definitions congruent? o Were key variables operationalized using the best possible method (e.g., interviews, observations, and so on) and with adequate justification? o Are specific instruments adequately described and were they good choices, given the study purpose, variables being studied, and the study population? o Does the report provide evidence that the data collection methods yielded data that were reliable and valid? **Anmerkung** Fragebögen warden beschrieben (p.2386f), Norvegische Version der Fragebögen wurden nicht auf die psychometrischen Eigenschaften getestet. Englische Version ist reliable und valide (p. 2386)	Teilweise
Procedures o If there was an intervention, is it adequately described, and was it rigor-ously developed and implemented? Did most participants allocated to the intervention group actually receive it? Is there evidence of intervention fi-delity? o Were data collected in a manner that minimized bias? Were the staff who collected data appropriately trained?	Keine Inter-vention

Results	
<u>Data analysis</u> o Were analyses undertaken to address each research question or test each hypothesis? o Were appropriate statistical methods used, given the level of measurement of the variables, number of groups being compared, and assumption of the tests? o Was the most powerful analytic method used (e.g., did the analysis help to control for confounding variables)? o Were Type I and Type II errors avoided or minimized? o In intervention studies, was an intention-to-treat analysis performed? o Were problems of missing values evaluated and adequately addressed?	Ja (p.2386)
<u>Findings</u> o Is information about statistical significance presented? Is information about effect size and precision of estimates (confidence intervals) presented? o Are the finding adequately summarized, with good use of tables and figures? o Are finding reported in a manner that facilitates a meta-analysis, and with sufficient information needed for EBP? **Anmerkung** Signifikanzniveau angeführt (p.2386), kein CI angeführt, Ergebnisse warden in Tabellen dargestellt (p.2387f)	Teilweise

Discussion	
<u>Interpretation of the findings</u> o Are all major findings interpreted and discussed within the context of prior research and/or the study's conceptual framework? o Are causal inferences, if any, justified? o Are interpretations well-founded and consistent with the study's limitations? o Does the report address the issue of the generalizability of the findings? **Anmerkung** Alle Ergebnisse warden interpretiert und diskutiert, (p.2388f), Limitatinen angeführt (p.2389f) Generalisierbarkeit der Studie wird in Frage gestellt (p.2389)	Teilweise
<u>Implications/recommendations</u> o Do the researchers discuss the implications of the study for clinical practice or further research – and are those implications reasonable and complete?	Ja (p.2390)

Global Issues	
Presentation o Is the report well-written, organized, and sufficiently detailed for critical analysis? o In intervention studies, is a CONSORT flow chart provides to show the flow of participants in the study? o Is the report written in a manner that makes the findings accessible to practicing nurses?	Ja
Researcher credibility o Do the researchers' clinical, substantive, or methodologic qualifications and experience enhance confidence in the findings and their interpretation?	Ja
Summary assessment o Despite any limitations, do the study findings appear to be valid, do you have confidence in the truth value of the results? o Does the study contribute any meaningful evidence that can be used in nursing practice or that is useful to the nursing discipline?	Ja

Lee et al., 2013

Title	
Is the title a good one, succinctly suggesting key variables and the study population?	Ja (p.140)

Abstract	
Does the abstract clearly and concisely summarize the main features of the report (problem, methods, results, conclusion)?	Ja (p.140)

Introduction	
Statement of the problem o Is the problem stated unambiguously, and is it easy to identify? o Does the problem statement build a cogent, persuasive argument for the new study? o Does the problem have significance for nursing? o Is there a good match between the research problem and the paradigm and methods used? Is a quantitative approach appropriate?	Ja (p.140)
Hypotheses or research question o Are research questions and/or hypotheses explicitly stated? If not, is their absence justified? o Are questions and hypotheses appropriately words, with clear specification of key variables and the study population? o Are the question/hypotheses consistent with the literature review and the conceptual framework?	Ja (p.141)
Literature review o Is the literature review up to date and based mainly on primary sources? o Does the review provide a state-of-the-art synthesis of evidence on the problem? o Does the literature review provide a sound basis for the new study?	Ja
Conceptual/theoretical framework o Are key concepts adequately defined conceptually? o Is there a conceptual/theoretical framework rationale, and/or map, and (if so) is it appropriate? If not, is the absence of one justified?	Nein

Method	
Protection of human rights o Were appropriate procedures used to safeguard the right of study participants? Was the study externally reviewed by an IRB/ethics review board? o Was the study designed to minimize risks and maximize benefits to participants?	Ja (p. 141)
Research designs o Was the most rigorous possible design used, given the study purpose? o Were appropriate comparisons made to enhance interpretability of the findings? o Was the number of data collection points appropriate? o Did the design minimize biases and threats to the internal, construct, and external validity of the study (e.g. was blinding used, was attrition minimized)?	Ja (p.141)
Population and sample o Is the population described? Is the sample described in sufficient detail? o Was the best possible sampling design used to enhance the sample's representativeness? Were sampling biases minimized? o Was the sample size adequate? Was a power analysis used to estimate sample size needs? **Anmerkung** Studienpopulation wird ausreichennd beschrieben (p. 142); k.A. ob Samplinggröße ausreichend war; Autoren wissen nicht wieviele Pflegeheime an dieser Befragung teilnahmen und ob es um Pflegeheime handelt, die sich auf Demenz spezialisiert haben, keine exakte Rücklaufquote bekannt (p. 145); keine Power-Analyse durchgeführt.	Teilweise
Data collection and measurements o Are the operational and conceptual definitions congruent? o Were key variables operationalized using the best possible method (e.g., interviews, observations, and so on) and with adequate justification? o Are specific instruments adequately described and were they good choices, given the study purpose, variables being studied, and the study population? o Does the report provide evidence that the data collection methods yielded data that were reliable and valid? **Anmerkung** Instrument wird beschrieben aber ist vorher nicht getestet worden (p.141), fehlende Angaben zu psychometrische Eigenschaften	Teilweise
Procedures o If there was an intervention, is it adequately described, and was it rigorously developed and implemented? Did most participants allocated to the intervention group actually receive it? Is there evidence of intervention fidelity? o Were data collected in a manner that minimized bias? Were the staff who collected data appropriately trained?	Keine Intervention

Results	
Data analysis	Ja (p.141f)
o Were analyses undertaken to address each research question or test each hypothesis?	
o Were appropriate statistical methods used, given the level of measurement of the variables, number of groups being compared, and assumption of the tests?	
o Was the most powerful analytic method used (e.g., did the analysis help to control for confounding variables)?	
o Were Type I and Type II errors avoided or minimized?	
o In intervention studies, was an intention-to-treat analysis performed?	
o Were problems of missing values evaluated and adequately addressed?	
Findings	Ja (p. 142f)
o Is information about statistical significance presented? Is information about effect size and precision of estimates (confidence intervals) presented?	
o Are the finding adequately summarized, with good use of tables and figures?	
o Are finding reported in a manner that facilitates a meta-analysis, and with sufficient information needed for EBP?	

Discussion	
Interpretation of the findings	Teilweise
o Are all major findings interpreted and discussed within the context of prior research and/or the study's conceptual framework?	
o Are causal inferences, if any, justified?	
o Are interpretations well-founded and consistent with the study's limitations?	
o Does the report address the issue of the generalizability of the findings?	
Anmerkung Alle Ergebnisse werden interpretiert und diskutiert, (p.144f), Limitationen werden angeführt (p.145), k.A. zur Generalisierbarkeit der Studie.	
Implications/recommendations	Teilweise
o Do the researchers discuss the implications of the study for clinical practice or further research – and are those implications reasonable and complete?	
Anmerkung Nicht ausführlich beschrieben	

Global Issues	
Presentation o Is the report well-written, organized, and sufficiently detailed for critical analysis? o In intervention studies, is a CONSORT flow chart provides to show the flow of participants in the study? o Is the report written in a manner that makes the findings accessible to practicing nurses?	Ja
Researcher credibility o Do the researchers' clinical, substantive, or methodologic qualifications and experience enhance confidence in the findings and their interpretation?	Ja
Summary assessment o Despite any limitations, do the study findings appear to be valid, do you have confidence in the truth value of the results? o Does the study contribute any meaningful evidence that can be used in nursing practice or that is useful to the nursing discipline?	Ja

Macdonald & Woods 2005

Title	
Is the title a good one, succinctly suggesting key variables and the study population?	Ja (p.383)

Abstract	
Does the abstract clearly and concisely summarize the main features of the report (problem, methods, results, conclusion)?	Ja (p.383)

Introduction	
Statement of the problem o Is the problem stated unambiguously, and is it easy to identify? o Does the problem statement build a cogent, persuasive argument for the new study? o Does the problem have significance for nursing? o Is there a good match between the research problem and the paradigm and methods used? Is a quantitative approach appropriate? **Anmerkung** Problem wird nicht ausführlich beschrieben, kurze Einleitung (p.384),	Teilweise
Hypotheses or research question o Are research questions and/or hypotheses explicitly stated? If not, is their absence justified? o Are questions and hypotheses appropriately words, with clear specification of key variables and the study population? o Are the question/hypotheses consistent with the literature review and the conceptual framework?	Ja (p.384)
Literature review o Is the literature review up to date and based mainly on primary sources? o Does the review provide a state-of-the-art synthesis of evidence on the problem? o Does the literature review provide a sound basis for the new study?	Ja
Conceptual/theoretical framework o Are key concepts adequately defined conceptually? o Is there a conceptual/theoretical framework rationale, and/or map, and (if so) is it appropriate? If not, is the absence of one justified?	Nein

Method	
Protection of human rights o Were appropriate procedures used to safeguard the right of study participants? Was the study externally reviewed by an IRB/ethics review board? o Was the study designed to minimize risks and maximize benefits to participants?	Ja (p.386)
Research designs o Was the most rigorous possible design used, given the study purpose? o Were appropriate comparisons made to enhance interpretability of the findings? o Was the number of data collection points appropriate? o Did the design minimize biases and threats to the internal, construct, and external validity of the study (e.g. was blinding used, was attrition minimized)? **Anmerkung** Forschugnsdesign angemessen, Zeitpunkt der Datenerhebung nicht optimal (p.390)	Teilweise
Population and sample o Is the population described? Is the sample described in sufficient detail? o Was the best possible sampling design used to enhance the sample's representativeness? Were sampling biases minimized? o Was the sample size adequate? Was a power analysis used to estimate sample size needs? **Anmerkung** Population unzureichend beschrieben (k.A. zu Alter, Geschlecht, Berufsgruppe), keine Power-Analyse	Teilweise
Data collection and measurements o Are the operational and conceptual definitions congruent? o Were key variables operationalized using the best possible method (e.g., interviews, observations, and so on) and with adequate justification? o Are specific instruments adequately described and were they good choices, given the study purpose, variables being studied, and the study population? o Does the report provide evidence that the data collection methods yielded data that were reliable and valid? **Anmerkung** Keine Definition von Demenz, ein Fragebogen (MMSE) wird nicht beschrieben, die anderen Instrumente werden beschrieben, psychometrische Eigenschaften angeführt (p.l384f)	Teilweise

Procedures	Keine Inter-vention
o If there was an intervention, is it adequately described, and was it rigorously developed and implemented? Did most participants allocated to the intervention group actually receive it? Is there evidence of intervention fidelity? o Were data collected in a manner that minimized bias? Were the staff who collected data appropriately trained?	

Results	
Data analysis	Ja (p.385f)
o Were analyses undertaken to address each research question or test each hypothesis? o Were appropriate statistical methods used, given the level of measurement of the variables, number of groups being compared, and assumption of the tests? o Was the most powerful analytic method used (e.g., did the analysis help to control for confounding variables)? o Were Type I and Type II errors avoided or minimized? o In intervention studies, was an intention-to-treat analysis performed? o Were problems of missing values evaluated and adequately addressed?	
Findings	Ja (p.386ff)
o Is information about statistical significance presented? Is information about effect size and precision of estimates (confidence intervals) presented? o Are the finding adequately summarized, with good use of tables and figures? o Are finding reported in a manner that facilitates a meta-analysis, and with sufficient information needed for EBP?	

Discussion	
Interpretation of the findings	Teilweise
o Are all major findings interpreted and discussed within the context of prior research and/or the study's conceptual framework? o Are causal inferences, if any, justified? o Are interpretations well-founded and consistent with the study's limitations? o Does the report address the issue of the generalizability of the findings? **Anmerkung** Es warden nicht alle Ergebnisse diskutiert, Generalisierbarkeit fraglich (p.390)	
Implications/recommendations	Nein
o Do the researchers discuss the implications of the study for clinical practice or further research – and are those implications reasonable and complete?	

Global Issues	
Presentation o Is the report well-written, organized, and sufficiently detailed for critical analysis? o In intervention studies, is a CONSORT flow chart provides to show the flow of participants in the study? o Is the report written in a manner that makes the findings accessible to practicing nurses?	Ja
Researcher credibility o Do the researchers' clinical, substantive, or methodologic qualifications and experience enhance confidence in the findings and their interpretation?	Ja
Summary assessment o Despite any limitations, do the study findings appear to be valid, do you have confidence in the truth value of the results? o Does the study contribute any meaningful evidence that can be used in nursing practice or that is useful to the nursing discipline?	Ja

Pellfolk et al., 2010

Title	
Is the title a good one, succinctly suggesting key variables and the study population? **Anmerkung** Setting fehlt, andere Variablen vorhanden (p.62)	Teilweise

Abstract	
Does the abstract clearly and concisely summarize the main features of the report (problem, methods, results, conclusion)?	Ja (p.62)

Introduction	
Statement of the problem o Is the problem stated unambiguously, and is it easy to identify? o Does the problem statement build a cogent, persuasive argument for the new study? o Does the problem have significance for nursing? o Is there a good match between the research problem and the paradigm and methods used? Is a quantitative approach appropriate?	Ja (p.62f)
Hypotheses or research question o Are research questions and/or hypotheses explicitly stated? If not, is their absence justified? o Are questions and hypotheses appropriately words, with clear specification of key variables and the study population? o Are the question/hypotheses consistent with the literature review and the conceptual framework? **Anmerkung** Keine Forschungsfrage oder Hypothese explizit angeführt, Forschungsziel ausführlich beschreiben (p.63)	Teilweise
Literature review o Is the literature review up to date and based mainly on primary sources? o Does the review provide a state-of-the-art synthesis of evidence on the problem? o Does the literature review provide a sound basis for the new study?	Ja
Conceptual/theoretical framework o Are key concepts adequately defined conceptually? o Is there a conceptual/theoretical framework rationale, and/or map, and (if so) is it appropriate? If not, is the absence of one justified?	Nein

Method	

Protection of human rights
 	
  o Were appropriate procedures used to safeguard the right of study partici-pants? Was the study externally reviewed by an IRB/ethics review board?
  o Was the study designed to minimize risks and maximize benefits to partici-pants?
	Ja (p.63)

Research designs
 	
  o Was the most rigorous possible design used, given the study purpose?
  o Were appropriate comparisons made to enhance interpretability of the findings?
  o Was the number of data collection points appropriate?
  o Did the design minimize biases and threats to the internal, construct, and external validity of the study (e.g. was blinding used, was attrition mini-mized)?
	Ja (p.63)

Population and sample
 	
  o Is the population described? Is the sample described in sufficient detail?
  o Was the best possible sampling design used to enhance the sample's rep-resentativeness? Were sampling biases minimized?
  o Was the sample size adequate? Was a power analysis used to estimate sample size needs?
 	
Anmerkung
Population wird beschrieben (p.64), Verteilung der Berufsgruppe fehlt, Power-Analye durchgeführt (p.66)
	Teilweise

Data collection and measurements
 	
  o Are the operational and conceptual definitions congruent?
  o Were key variables operationalized using the best possible method (e.g., interviews, observations, and so on) and with adequate justification?
  o Are specific instruments adequately described and were they good choices, given the study purpose, variables being studied, and the study population?
  o Does the report provide evidence that the data collection methods yielded data that were reliable and valid?
	Ja (p.64ff)

Procedures
 	
  o If there was an intervention, is it adequately described, and was it rigor-ously developed and implemented? Did most participants allocated to the intervention group actually receive it? Is there evidence of intervention fi-delity?
  o Were data collected in a manner that minimized bias? Were the staff who collected data appropriately trained?
 	
Anmerkung
Intervention wird beschrieben (p.64), Assessment für die Bewohner führten Pflegepersonen aus, Fragebogen könnte zu früh oder zu spat ausgefüllt worden sein (p.68)
	Teilweise

Results	
Data analysis	Ja (p.66f)
o Were analyses undertaken to address each research question or test each hypothesis? o Were appropriate statistical methods used, given the level of measurement of the variables, number of groups being compared, and assumption of the tests? o Was the most powerful analytic method used (e.g., did the analysis help to control for confounding variables)? o Were Type I and Type II errors avoided or minimized? o In intervention studies, was an intention-to-treat analysis performed? o Were problems of missing values evaluated and adequately addressed?	
Findings	Ja (p.64ff)
o Is information about statistical significance presented? Is information about effect size and precision of estimates (confidence intervals) presented? o Are the finding adequately summarized, with good use of tables and figures? o Are finding reported in a manner that facilitates a meta-analysis, and with sufficient information needed for EBP?	

Discussion	
Interpretation of the findings	Teilweise
o Are all major findings interpreted and discussed within the context of prior research and/or the study's conceptual framework? o Are causal inferences, if any, justified? o Are interpretations well-founded and consistent with the study's limitations? o Does the report address the issue of the generalizability of the findings? **Anmerkung** Alle Ergebnisse werden interpretiert und diskutiert, (p.67f)), Limitatinen angeführt (p.68), k.A. zur Generalisierbarkeit der Studie	
Implications/recommendations	Ja (p.68)
o Do the researchers discuss the implications of the study for clinical practice or further research – and are those implications reasonable and complete?	

Global Issues	
Presentation o Is the report well-written, organized, and sufficiently detailed for critical analysis? o In intervention studies, is a CONSORT flow chart provides to show the flow of participants in the study? o Is the report written in a manner that makes the findings accessible to practicing nurses?	Ja
Researcher credibility o Do the researchers' clinical, substantive, or methodologic qualifications and experience enhance confidence in the findings and their interpretation?	Ja
Summary assessment o Despite any limitations, do the study findings appear to be valid, do you have confidence in the truth value of the results? o Does the study contribute any meaningful evidence that can be used in nursing practice or that is useful to the nursing discipline?	Ja

Robinson et al., 2014

Title	
Is the title a good one, succinctly suggesting key variables and the study population?	Ja (p.158)

Abstract	
Does the abstract clearly and concisely summarize the main features of the report (problem, methods, results, conclusion)?	Ja (p.158)

Introduction	
Statement of the problem o Is the problem stated unambiguously, and is it easy to identify? o Does the problem statement build a cogent, persuasive argument for the new study? o Does the problem have significance for nursing? o Is there a good match between the research problem and the paradigm and methods used? Is a quantitative approach appropriate?	Ja (p.158f)
Hypotheses or research question o Are research questions and/or hypotheses explicitly stated? If not, is their absence justified? o Are questions and hypotheses appropriately words, with clear specification of key variables and the study population? o Are the question/hypotheses consistent with the literature review and the conceptual framework? **Anmerkung** Keine Forschungsfrage oder Hypothese formuliert, Forschungsziel vorhanden – alle Variablen vorhanden (p.584)	Teilweise
Literature review o Is the literature review up to date and based mainly on primary sources? o Does the review provide a state-of-the-art synthesis of evidence on the problem? o Does the literature review provide a sound basis for the new study?	Ja
Conceptual/theoretical framework o Are key concepts adequately defined conceptually? o Is there a conceptual/theoretical framework rationale, and/or map, and (if so) is it appropriate? If not, is the absence of one justified?	Nein

Method	
Protection of human rights o Were appropriate procedures used to safeguard the right of study participants? Was the study externally reviewed by an IRB/ethics review board? o Was the study designed to minimize risks and maximize benefits to participants?	Ja (p. 159)
Research designs o Was the most rigorous possible design used, given the study purpose? o Were appropriate comparisons made to enhance interpretability of the findings? o Was the number of data collection points appropriate? o Did the design minimize biases and threats to the internal, construct, and external validity of the study (e.g. was blinding used, was attrition minimized)?	Ja (p.159)
Population and sample o Is the population described? Is the sample described in sufficient detail? o Was the best possible sampling design used to enhance the sample's representativeness? Were sampling biases minimized? o Was the sample size adequate? Was a power analysis used to estimate sample size needs? **Anmerkung** Studienpopulation wird ausreichennd beschrieben (p. 160f); möglicher Sampling-Bias: nicht alle Pflegepersonen erreicht (p. 159); k.A. ob Samplinggröße ausreichend war; keine Power-Analyse durchgeführt	Teilweise
Data collection and measurements o Are the operational and conceptual definitions congruent? o Were key variables operationalized using the best possible method (e.g., interviews, observations, and so on) and with adequate justification? o Are specific instruments adequately described and were they good choices, given the study purpose, variables being studied, and the study population? o Does the report provide evidence that the data collection methods yielded data that were reliable and valid?	Ja (p.160)
Procedures o If there was an intervention, is it adequately described, and was it rigorously developed and implemented? Did most participants allocated to the intervention group actually receive it? Is there evidence of intervention fidelity? o Were data collected in a manner that minimized bias? Were the staff who collected data appropriately trained?	Keine Intervention

Results	
<u>Data analysis</u>	Ja (p.160)
o Were analyses undertaken to address each research question or test each hypothesis? o Were appropriate statistical methods used, given the level of measurement of the variables, number of groups being compared, and assumption of the tests? o Was the most powerful analytic method used (e.g., did the analysis help to control for confounding variables)? o Were Type I and Type II errors avoided or minimized? o In intervention studies, was an intention-to-treat analysis performed? o Were problems of missing values evaluated and adequately addressed?	
<u>Findings</u>	Teilweise
o Is information about statistical significance presented? Is information about effect size and precision of estimates (confidence intervals) presented? o Are the finding adequately summarized, with good use of tables and figures? o Are finding reported in a manner that facilitates a meta-analysis, and with sufficient information needed for EBP? **Anmerkung** Signifikanzniveau angeführt (p.161f), kein CI angeführt, Ergebnisse werden in Tabellen dargestellt (p161f)	

Discussion	
<u>Interpretation of the findings</u>	Teilweise
o Are all major findings interpreted and discussed within the context of prior research and/or the study's conceptual framework? o Are causal inferences, if any, justified? o Are interpretations well-founded and consistent with the study's limitations? o Does the report address the issue of the generalizability of the findings? **Anmerkung** Alle Ergebnisse warden interpretiert und diskutiert, (p.161ff), k.A. zu Limitationen und Generalisierbarkeit der Studie.	
<u>Implications/recommendations</u>	Ja (p. 163)
o Do the researchers discuss the implications of the study for clinical practice or further research – and are those implications reasonable and complete?	

Global Issues	
Presentation o Is the report well-written, organized, and sufficiently detailed for critical analysis? o In intervention studies, is a CONSORT flow chart provides to show the flow of participants in the study? o Is the report written in a manner that makes the findings accessible to practicing nurses?	Ja
Researcher credibility o Do the researchers' clinical, substantive, or methodologic qualifications and experience enhance confidence in the findings and their interpretation?	Ja
Summary assessment o Despite any limitations, do the study findings appear to be valid, do you have confidence in the truth value of the results? o Does the study contribute any meaningful evidence that can be used in nursing practice or that is useful to the nursing discipline?	Ja

Zimmerman et al., 2005a

Title	
Is the title a good one, succinctly suggesting key variables and the study population?	Ja (p.96)

Abstract	
Does the abstract clearly and concisely summarize the main features of the report (problem, methods, results, conclusion)?	Ja (p.96)

Introduction	
Statement of the problem o Is the problem stated unambiguously, and is it easy to identify? o Does the problem statement build a cogent, persuasive argument for the new study? o Does the problem have significance for nursing? o Is there a good match between the research problem and the paradigm and methods used? Is a quantitative approach appropriate?	Ja (p.96f)
Hypotheses or research question o Are research questions and/or hypotheses explicitly stated? If not, is their absence justified? o Are questions and hypotheses appropriately words, with clear specification of key variables and the study population? o Are the question/hypotheses consistent with the literature review and the conceptual framework? **Anmerkung** Keine Forschungsfrage oder Hypothese explizit angeführt, Forschungsziel ausführlich beschreiben (p.97)	Teilweise
Literature review o Is the literature review up to date and based mainly on primary sources? o Does the review provide a state-of-the-art synthesis of evidence on the problem? o Does the literature review provide a sound basis for the new study?	Ja
Conceptual/theoretical framework o Are key concepts adequately defined conceptually? o Is there a conceptual/theoretical framework rationale, and/or map, and (if so) is it appropriate? If not, is the absence of one justified?	Ja (p.97)

Method	
Protection of human rights o Were appropriate procedures used to safeguard the right of study participants? Was the study externally reviewed by an IRB/ethics review board? o Was the study designed to minimize risks and maximize benefits to participants?	Ja (p.97)
Research designs o Was the most rigorous possible design used, given the study purpose? o Were appropriate comparisons made to enhance interpretability of the findings? o Was the number of data collection points appropriate? o Did the design minimize biases and threats to the internal, construct, and external validity of the study (e.g. was blinding used, was attrition minimized)?	Ja (p.97)
Population and sample o Is the population described? Is the sample described in sufficient detail? o Was the best possible sampling design used to enhance the sample's representativeness? Were sampling biases minimized? o Was the sample size adequate? Was a power analysis used to estimate sample size needs? **Anmerkung** Studienpopulation wird ausreichend beschrieben (p.97), k.A. zur Power-Analyse, k.A zur Fragebogenerhebung	Teilweise
Data collection and measurements o Are the operational and conceptual definitions congruent? o Were key variables operationalized using the best possible method (e.g., interviews, observations, and so on) and with adequate justification? o Are specific instruments adequately described and were they good choices, given the study purpose, variables being studied, and the study population? o Does the report provide evidence that the data collection methods yielded data that were reliable and valid? **Anmerkung** Keine Definition zu Demenz, Fragebögen werden kurz erläutert (p.98), unvollständige pychometrische Eigenschaften, Interne Konsistenz wurde berechnet (p.100)	Teilweise
Procedures o If there was an intervention, is it adequately described, and was it rigorously developed and implemented? Did most participants allocated to the intervention group actually receive it? Is there evidence of intervention fidelity? o Were data collected in a manner that minimized bias? Were the staff who collected data appropriately trained? Anmerkung	Teilweise

Results	
<u>Data analysis</u>	Ja (p.98f)
o Were analyses undertaken to address each research question or test each hypothesis? o Were appropriate statistical methods used, given the level of measurement of the variables, number of groups being compared, and assumption of the tests? o Was the most powerful analytic method used (e.g., did the analysis help to control for confounding variables)? o Were Type I and Type II errors avoided or minimized? o In intervention studies, was an intention-to-treat analysis performed? o Were problems of missing values evaluated and adequately addressed?	
<u>Findings</u>	Teilweise
o Is information about statistical significance presented? Is information about effect size and precision of estimates (confidence intervals) presented? o Are the finding adequately summarized, with good use of tables and figures? o Are finding reported in a manner that facilitates a meta-analysis, and with sufficient information needed for EBP? **Anmerkung** p-Werte werden angeführt, keine CI, Tabellen (99ff)	

Discussion	
<u>Interpretation of the findings</u>	Teilweise
o Are all major findings interpreted and discussed within the context of prior research and/or the study's conceptual framework? o Are causal inferences, if any, justified? o Are interpretations well-founded and consistent with the study's limitations? o Does the report address the issue of the generalizability of the findings? **Anmerkung** Alle Ergebnisse warden interpretiert und diskutiert, (p.304f)), Limitatinen angeführt (p.305f), Generalisierbarkeit wird in Frage gestellt (p.104)	
<u>Implications/recommendations</u>	Ja (p.103f)
o Do the researchers discuss the implications of the study for clinical practice or further research – and are those implications reasonable and complete?	

Global Issues	
Presentation o Is the report well-written, organized, and sufficiently detailed for critical analysis? o In intervention studies, is a CONSORT flow chart provides to show the flow of participants in the study? o Is the report written in a manner that makes the findings accessible to practicing nurses?	Ja
Researcher credibility o Do the researchers' clinical, substantive, or methodologic qualifications and experience enhance confidence in the findings and their interpretation?	Ja
Summary assessment o Despite any limitations, do the study findings appear to be valid, do you have confidence in the truth value of the results? o Does the study contribute any meaningful evidence that can be used in nursing practice or that is useful to the nursing discipline?	Ja

Zimmermann et al., 2010

Title	
Is the title a good one, succinctly suggesting key variables and the study population?	Ja (p.83)

Abstract	
Does the abstract clearly and concisely summarize the main features of the report (problem, methods, results, conclusion)? **Anmerkung** Keine Problembeschreibung, andere Variablen vorhanden (p.83)	Teilweies

Introduction	
Statement of the problem o Is the problem stated unambiguously, and is it easy to identify? o Does the problem statement build a cogent, persuasive argument for the new study? o Does the problem have significance for nursing? o Is there a good match between the research problem and the paradigm and methods used? Is a quantitative approach appropriate?	Ja (p.83)
Hypotheses or research question o Are research questions and/or hypotheses explicitly stated? If not, is their absence justified? o Are questions and hypotheses appropriately words, with clear specification of key variables and the study population? o Are the question/hypotheses consistent with the literature review and the conceptual framework? **Anmerkung** Keine Forschungsfrage oder Hypothese explizit angeführt, Forschungsziel beschreiben (p.84)	Teilweise
Literature review o Is the literature review up to date and based mainly on primary sources? o Does the review provide a state-of-the-art synthesis of evidence on the problem? o Does the literature review provide a sound basis for the new study?	Ja
Conceptual/theoretical framework o Are key concepts adequately defined conceptually? o Is there a conceptual/theoretical framework rationale, and/or map, and (if so) is it appropriate? If not, is the absence of one justified?	Ja (p.84)

Method	
Protection of human rights o Were appropriate procedures used to safeguard the right of study participants? Was the study externally reviewed by an IRB/ethics review board? o Was the study designed to minimize risks and maximize benefits to participants?	Ja (p.85)
Research designs o Was the most rigorous possible design used, given the study purpose? o Were appropriate comparisons made to enhance interpretability of the findings? o Was the number of data collection points appropriate? o Did the design minimize biases and threats to the internal, construct, and external validity of the study (e.g. was blinding used, was attrition minimized)?	Ja (p.84f)
Population and sample o Is the population described? Is the sample described in sufficient detail? o Was the best possible sampling design used to enhance the sample's representativeness? Were sampling biases minimized? o Was the sample size adequate? Was a power analysis used to estimate sample size needs? **Anmerkung** Studienpopulation wird ausreichend beschrieben (p.89), k.A. zur Power-Analyse	Teilweise
Data collection and measurements o Are the operational and conceptual definitions congruent? o Were key variables operationalized using the best possible method (e.g., interviews, observations, and so on) and with adequate justification? o Are specific instruments adequately described and were they good choices, given the study purpose, variables being studied, and the study population? o Does the report provide evidence that the data collection methods yielded data that were reliable and valid? **Anmerkung** Keine Definition zu Demenz, Fragebögen warden kurz erläutert (p.98), k.A. zu pychometrische Eigenschaften	Teilweise
Procedures o If there was an intervention, is it adequately described, and was it rigorously developed and implemented? Did most participants allocated to the intervention group actually receive it? Is there evidence of intervention fidelity? o Were data collected in a manner that minimized bias? Were the staff who collected data appropriately trained?	Ja (p.87f)

Results	
Data analysis o Were analyses undertaken to address each research question or test each hypothesis? o Were appropriate statistical methods used, given the level of measurement of the variables, number of groups being compared, and assumption of the tests? o Was the most powerful analytic method used (e.g., did the analysis help to control for confounding variables)? o Were Type I and Type II errors avoided or minimized? o In intervention studies, was an intention-to-treat analysis performed? o Were problems of missing values evaluated and adequately addressed?	Ja (p.98f)
Findings o Is information about statistical significance presented? Is information about effect size and precision of estimates (confidence intervals) presented? o Are the finding adequately summarized, with good use of tables and figures? o Are finding reported in a manner that facilitates a meta-analysis, and with sufficient information needed for EBP? **Anmerkung** p-Werte werden angeführt, keine CI, Tabellen (84ff)	Teilweise

Discussion	
Interpretation of the findings o Are all major findings interpreted and discussed within the context of prior research and/or the study's conceptual framework? o Are causal inferences, if any, justified? o Are interpretations well-founded and consistent with the study's limitations? o Does the report address the issue of the generalizability of the findings? **Anmerkung** Alle Ergebnisse warden interpretiert und diskutiert, (p.304f)), Limitatinen angeführt (p.305f), k.A zur Generalisierbarkeit	Teilweise
Implications/recommendations o Do the researchers discuss the implications of the study for clinical practice or further research – and are those implications reasonable and complete?	Ja (p.103f)

Global Issues	
Presentation ○ Is the report well-written, organized, and sufficiently detailed for critical analysis? ○ In intervention studies, is a CONSORT flow chart provides to show the flow of participants in the study? ○ Is the report written in a manner that makes the findings accessible to practicing nurses?	Ja
Researcher credibility ○ Do the researchers' clinical, substantive, or methodologic qualifications and experience enhance confidence in the findings and their interpretation?	Ja
Summary assessment ○ Despite any limitations, do the study findings appear to be valid, do you have confidence in the truth value of the results? ○ Does the study contribute any meaningful evidence that can be used in nursing practice or that is useful to the nursing discipline?	Ja

8. Anhang 3: Bewertung der qualitativen Studien

Chang et al., 2009

Title	
Is the title a good one, succinctly suggesting key phenomenon and the group or community under study?	Ja (p.41)

Abstract	
Does the abstract clearly and concisely summarize the main features of the report?	Ja (p.41f)

Introduction	
Statement of the problem o Is the problem stated unambiguously, and is it easy to identify? o Does the problem statement build a cogent, persuasive argument for the new study? o Does the problem have significance for nursing? o Is there a good match between the research problem and the one hand and the paradigm, tradition, and methods on the other?	Ja (p.42)
Hypotheses or research question o Are research questions explicitly stated? If not, is their absence justified? o Are the questions consistent with the study's philosophical basis, underlying tradition, conceptual framework, or ideological orientation? **Anmerkung** Keine Forschungsfrage/n formuliert, Ziel wurde formuliert	Teilweise
Literature review o Does the report adequately summarize the existing body of knowledge related to the problem or phenomenon of interest? o Does the literature review provide a solid basis for the new study?	Ja (p.42)
Conceptual underpinnings o Are key concepts adequately defined conceptually? o Is the philosophical basis, underlying tradition, conceptual framework, or ideological orientation made explicit and is it appropriate for the problem? **Anmerkung** Keine konzeptueller Rahmen vorhanden, Defintion von Demenz gegeben (p.42), Beschreibungen der Fokusgruppen vorhanden (p.43)	Teilweise

Method	
Protection of human rights o Were appropriate procedures used to safeguard the right of study participants? Was the study subject to external review? o Was the study designed to minimize risks and maximize benefits to participants?	Ja (p.43)
Research designs and research tradition o Is the identified research tradition (if any) congruent with the methods used to collect and analyze data? o Was an adequate amount of time spent in the field or with study participants? o Did the design unfold in the field, giving researchers opportunities to capitalize on early understandings? o Was there evidence of reflexivity in the design? o Was there an adequate number of contacts with study participants?	Ja (p.42f)
Sample and setting o Was the group or population of interest adequately described? Were the setting and sample described in sufficient detail? o Was the approach used to gain access to the site or to recruit participants appropriate? o Was the best possible method of sampling used to enhance information richness and address the needs of the study? o Was the sample size adequate? Was saturation achieved? **Anmerkung** Studienpopulation ausreichend beschrieben (p.43), Samplingröße zu klein (p.45)	Teilweise
Data collection o Were the methods of gathering data appropriate? Were data gathered through two or more methods to achieve triangulation? o Did the researcher ask the right questions or make the right observations, and were they recorded in an appropriate fashion? o Was a sufficient amount of data gathered? Was the data of sufficient depth and richness?	Ja (p.43)
Procedures o Were data collection and recording procedures adequately described and do they appear appropriate? o Were data collected in a manner that minimized bias or behavioral distortions? Were the staff who collected data appropriately trained?	Ja (p.43)
Enhancement of rigor o Were methods used to enhance the trustworthiness of the data (and analysis), and was the description of those methods adequate? o Were the methods used to enhance credibility appropriate and sufficient? o Did the researcher document research procedures and decision processes sufficiently that findings are auditable and confirmable?	Ja (p.43)

Results	
<u>Data analysis</u> o Were the data management (e.g., coding) and data analysis methods suffiently described? o Was the data analysis strategy compatible with the research tradition and with the nature and type of data gathered? o Did the analysis yield an appropriate "product" (e.g., a theory, taconomy, thematic pattern, etc.)? o Did the analytic procedures suggest the possibility of biases?	Ja (p.43)
<u>Finding</u> o Were the findings effectively summarized with good use of excerpts and supporting arguments? o Do the the adequately capture the meaning of data? Does, it appear that the researcher satisfactorily conceptualized the themes or pattern in the data? o Did the analysis yield an insightful, provocative, and meaningful picture of the phenomenon under investigation?	Ja (p.43ff)
<u>Theoretical intergration</u> o Are the themes or patterns logically connected to each other to form a convincing and integrated whole? o Were figures, maps, or models uses effectively to summarize conceptualization? o If a conceptual framework or ideological orientation guided the study, are the thes or pattern linked to it in a cogent manner? **Anmerkung** Logischer Aufbau, keine Abbildungen/Modelle vorhanden	Teilweise

Discussion	
<u>Interpretation of the findings</u> o Are the finding interpreted within an appropriate frame of reference? o Are major finding interpreted and discussed within the context of prior studies? o Are the interpretations consistent with the study's limitation? o Does the report address the issue of the transferability of the finding?	Ja (p.45f)
<u>Implications/recommendations</u> o Do the researchers discuss the implications of the study for clinical practice or furtherinquiry – and are those implications reasonable and complete?	Ja (p.46)

Global Issues	
Presentation o Is the report well-written, organized, and sufficiently detailed for critical analysis? o Was the description of the methods, findings, and interpretations sufficiently rich and vivid?	Ja
Researcher credibility o Do the researchers' clinical, substantive, or methodologic qualifications and experience enhance confidence in the findings and their interpretation?	Ja
Summary assessment o Do the study findings appear to be trustworthy do you have confidence in the truth value of the results? o Does the study contribute any meaningful evidence that can be used in nursing practice or that is useful to the nursing discipline?	Ja

Furåker & Nilsson 2009

Title	
Is the title a good one, succinctly suggesting key phenomenon and the group or community under study?	Ja (p.146)

Abstract	
Does the abstract clearly and concisely summarize the main features of the report?	Ja (p.146)

Introduction	
Statement of the problem o Is the problem stated unambiguously, and is it easy to identify? o Does the problem statement build a cogent, persuasive argument for the new study? o Does the problem have significance for nursing? o Is there a good match between the research problem and the one hand and the paradigm, tradition, and methods on the other?	Ja (p.146f)
Hypotheses or research question o Are research questions explicitly stated? If not, is their absence justified? o Are the questions consistent with the study's philosophical basis, underlying tradition, conceptual framework, or ideological orientation? **Anmerkung** Keine Forschungsfrage/n, Ziel wurde formuliert (p.146)	Teilweise
Literature review o Does the report adequately summarize the existing body of knowledge related to the problem or phenomenon of interest? o Does the literature review provide a solid basis for the new study?	Ja (p.146f)
Conceptual underpinnings o Are key concepts adequately defined conceptually? o Is the philosophical basis, underlying tradition, conceptual framework, or ideological orientation made explicit and is it appropriate for the problem? **Anmerkung** Schlüsselkonzepte warden formuliert (p.147), kein konzeptueller Rahmen	Teilweise

121

Method	
Protection of human rights o Were appropriate procedures used to safeguard the right of study partici- pants? Was the study subject to external review? o Was the study designed to minimize risks and maximize benefits to partici- pants? **Anmerkung** Über Freiwilligkeit und Rechte aufgeklärt (p.148), k.A. zum externen Reviewe	Teilweise
Research designs and research tradition o Is the identified research tradition (if any) congruent with the methods used to collect and analyze data? o Was an adequate amount of time spent in the field or with study partici- pants? o Did the design unfold in the field, giving researchers opportunities to capi- talize on early understandings? o Was there evidence of reflexivity in the design? o Was there an adequate number of contacts with study participants?	Ja (p.147)
Sample and setting o Was the group or population of interest adequately described? Were the setting and sample described in sufficient detail? o Was the approach used to gain access to the site or to recruit participants appropriate? o Was the best possible method of sampling used to enhance information richness and address the needs of the study? o Was the sample size adequate? Was saturation achieved? **Anmerkung** Studienpopulation ausreichend beschrieben (p.147), k.A. zur Samplinggröße	Teilweise
Data collection o Were the methods of gathering data appropriate? Were data gathered through two or more methods to achieve triangulation? o Did the researcher ask the right questions or make the right observations, and were they recorded in an appropriate fashion? o Was a sufficient amount of data gathered? Was the data of sufficient depth and richness?	Ja (147)
Procedures o Were data collection and recording procedures adequately described and do they appear appropriate? o Were data collected in a manner that minimized bias or behavioral distor- tions? Were the staff who collected data appropriately trained? **Anmerkung** Prozedere ausreichend beschrieben (p.147f), Interviews wurden mit interess- ierten TeilnehmerInnen geführt (p.148) –Bias-Gefahr	Teilweise

Enhancement of rigor	Ja (p.148)
o Were methods used to enhance the trustworthiness of the data (and analysis), and was the description of those methods adequate? o Were the methods used to enhance credibility appropriate and sufficient? o Did the researcher document research procedures and decision processes sufficiently that findings are auditable and confirmable?	

Results	
Data analysis	Ja (p.148)
o Were the data management (e.g., coding) and data analysis methods suffiently described? o ·Was the data analysis strategy compatible with the research tradition and with the nature and type of data gathered? o Did the analysis yield an appropriate "product" (e.g., a theory, taconomy, thematic pattern, etc.)? o Did the analytic procedures suggest the possibility of biases?	
Finding	Ja (p.148ff)
o Were the findings effectively summarized with good use of excerpts and supporting arguments? o Do the the adequately capture the meaning of data? Does, it appear that the researcher satisfactorily conceptualized the themes or pattern in the data? o Did the analysis yield an insightful, provocative, and meaningful picture of the phenomenon under investigation?	
Theoretical intergration	Teilweise
o Are the themes or patterns logically connected to each other to form a convincing and integrated whole? o Were figures, maps, or models uses effectively to summarize conceptualization? o If a conceptual framework or ideological orientation guided the study, are the thes or pattern linked to it in a cogent manner? **Anmerkung** Logischer Aufbau (p.148ff), keine Abbildungen/Modelle vorhanden	

Discussion	
Interpretation of the findings	Teilweise
o Are the finding interpreted within an appropriate frame of reference? o Are major finding interpreted and discussed within the context of prior studies? o Are the interpretations consistent with the study's limitation? o Does the report address the issue of the transferability of the finding? **Anmerkung** Ergebnisse werden mit anderen Studienv verglichen (p.150f), k.A. zu Limitationen	

Discussion	
Implications/recommendations o Do the researchers discuss the implications of the study for clinical practice or furtherinquiry – and are those implications reasonable and complete?	Ja (p.151)

Global Issues	
Presentation o Is the report well-written, organized, and sufficiently detailed for critical analysis? o Was the description of the methods, findings, and interpretations sufficiently rich and vivid?	Ja
Researcher credibility o Do the researchers' clinical, substantive, or methodologic qualifications and experience enhance confidence in the findings and their interpretation?	Ja
Summary assessment o Do the study findings appear to be trustworthy do you have confidence in the truth value of the results? o Does the study contribute any meaningful evidence that can be used in nursing practice or that is useful to the nursing discipline?	Ja

Printed in the United States
By Bookmasters